Name:_____ Date(s): _____

If you are willing to invest the time and effort, we anticipate that this course experience will be most rewarding and beneficial. Before beginning this course, complete the Pre-course Assessment column. At the end of the course, come back and fill out the Post-course Assessment; see the progress you have made!

	PRE-COURSE ASSESSMENT	POST-COURSE ASSESSMENT
How do you define stress?		
What causes stress?		
What happens if you have too much stress?		
What is the current cause of stress in your life?		
On a scale of 1 to 5 what is your current stress level?	LOW 1 2 3 4 5 HIGH	LOW 1 2 3 4 5 HIGH
How does this stress affect your daily life?		
Are you currently experiencing any physical symptoms of stress (tight muscles, sickness, etc)?		
What stress management techniques are most helpful in managing the stress in your life?		
Yogic Breathing	Have you ever tried breathing techniques as a way to alleviate stress? What is your impression of this technique?	On a scale of 1 to 5, how effective was this technique in helping you to manage your stress? LOW 1 2 3 4 5 HIGH How will you incorporate this technique into your daily life?

D1455891

	PRE-COURSE ASSESSMENT	POST-COURSE ASSESSMENT
Progressive Muscle Relaxation	Have you ever tried Progressive Muscle Relaxation as a way to alleviate stress? What is your impression of this technique?	On a scale of 1 to 5, how effective was this technique in helping you to manage your stress? LOW 1 2 3 4 5 HIGH How will you incorporate this technique into your daily life?
Autogenic Training	Have you ever tried Autogenic Training as a way to alleviate stress? What is your impression of this technique?	On a scale of 1 to 5, how effective was this technique in helping you to manage your stress? LOW 1 2 3 4 5 HIGH How will you incorporate this technique into your daily life?
Visual Imagery	Have you ever tried Visual Imagery as a way to alleviate stress? What is your impression of this technique?	On a scale of 1 to 5, how effective was this technique in helping you to manage your stress? LOW 1 2 3 4 5 HIGH How will you incorporate this technique into your daily life?
How many times a week do you exercise?		
What does your typical diet consist of?		
How do you manage your time?		
Do you find yourself rushing to class or appointments?		
What positive life changes will you make to help manage your stress?		

SIXTH EDITION

PRACTICAL STRESS MANAGEMENT

A COMPREHENSIVE WORKBOOK

JOHN A. ROMAS
Minnesota State University, Mankato

MANOJ SHARMA
University of Cincinnati

PEARSON

BOSTON   COLUMBUS   INDIANAPOLIS   NEW YORK   SAN FRANCISCO
UPPER SADDLE RIVER   AMSTERDAM   CAPE TOWN   DUBAI   LONDON   MADRID
MILAN   MUNICH   PARIS   MONTRÉAL   TORONTO   DELHI   MEXICO CITY
SÃO PAULO   SYDNEY   HONG KONG   SEOUL   SINGAPORE   TAIPEI   TOKYO

Executive Editor: Sandra Lindelof
Editorial Manager: Susan Malloy
Project Manager: Carol Traver/Azimuth Publisher Services
Editorial Assistant: Briana Verdugo
Executive Marketing Manager: Neena Bali
Senior Managing Editor: Deborah Cogan

Production Project Manager: Dorothy Cox
Senior Manufacturing Buyer: Stacey Weinberger
Production Management and Composition: PreMediaGlobal
Interior Designer: Seventeenth Street Studios
Cover Designer: Riezebos Holzbaur Group
Cover Photo: Noah Clayton/Getty Images

ISBN 10: 0-321-88364-0
ISBN 13: 978-0-321-88364-3

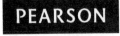

www.pearsonhighered.com

5 6 7 8 9 10—V0UD—20 19 18 17 16

MAY OUR
CHILDREN ASPIRE
TO BECOME THE
ONES THEY DREAM
TO BE AND BRING
SUNSHINE TO
THEMSELVES
AS WELL AS
OTHERS

To Judi, Jennifer,
and Mom and Dad
——J. A. ROMAS

To Mummy, Daddy, and Guruji
and Sulekha, Ankita, and Malvika
——M. SHARMA

In Fond Memory of Dr. E.J. McClendon
Scholar, Mentor, Friend

Brief Contents

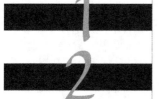
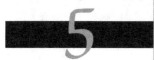

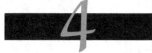
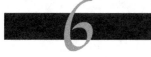
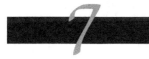
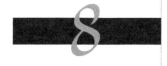

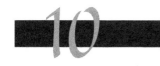
v

Detailed Contents

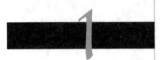
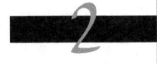

RELAXATION 55

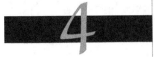

EFFECTIVE COMMUNICATION 80

MANAGING ANGER AND RESOLVING CONFLICTS 99

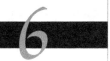

6 COPING WITH ANXIETY 123

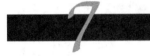

7 EATING BEHAVIORS FOR HEALTHY LIFESTYLES 147

8 REGULAR PHYSICAL ACTIVITY AND EXERCISE 174

9 EFFICIENT TIME MANAGEMENT AND SOUND FINANCIAL MANAGEMENT 189

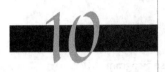

IMPLEMENTING A STRESS REDUCTION PLAN 211

Preface

Since its first publication in 1995, this workbook has sold over 15,000 copies. We have been extremely pleased with this response and hope that this edition will continue to receive the same love, support, and admiration in the coming years. This workbook is not only popular in the United States and Canada but also has readers from other countries. This popularity reaffirms that the techniques discussed in this workbook are quite universal and not confined to any one region of the world. We are hopeful that the new readers of this workbook will continue to grow, learn, and apply the techniques presented to achieve greater satisfaction in their lives.

In the first edition of this workbook, we presented a pragmatic approach to stress management in a simple language. Our focus was on practicality and based upon scientific research and documented techniques. We introduced Worksheets, Thoughts for Reflection, Stress Management Principles, and Summary Points for each chapter. We blended thoughts—contemporary and old, Eastern and Western, medical and behavioral, traditional and scientific. Our aim was to help readers lead balanced, peaceful, and satisfying lives. All these features were well received by our readers from both academic and nonacademic settings.

Throughout the revisions of the workbook, we have maintained the user-friendly and pragmatic approach and continued with the "cafeteria" approach, allowing readers to pick and choose the techniques that they wanted to adopt. We have continued to make improvements and enhancements, with the inclusion of new topics, creation of PowerPoint slides for instructors, and ongoing updates.

In the *sixth edition* of this workbook, we have continued with the remarkable features of this book that include:

○ Using the approach of a workbook format with practical worksheets.

○ Introducing a variety of methods to combat stress that can be handpicked by the reader to suit his or her needs.

○ Organizing the materials in such a way that they can be delivered in both quarter and semester courses.

○ Emphasizing a preventive approach that is appealing to readers from all walks of life.

○ Promoting self-reliance in readers so that the techniques described in this workbook can be mastered without any external help.

○ Facilitating positive behavior changes in readers so that they can derive greater contentment in their lives.

Some specific changes that we have made in the sixth edition include:

○ Introducing a website (www.pearsonhighered.com/romas) at which students can access MP3 files of the audio files guiding them through relaxation techniques of yogic breathing (*pranayama*), progressive muscle relaxation, autogenic training, and visual imagery. Students can now use these techniques with whatever electronic device they choose.

○ Adding the worksheets and pre- and post-course self-assessment to the same website, giving students the opportunity to download them if that is their preference.

○ Providing the pre- and post-course assessment found at the front of the book on heavier paper, making it more useful for students throughout the quarter or semester.

○ Updating the references and websites in all the chapters.

○ Making the worksheets more user friendly in all the chapters.

○ Introducing information on sense of coherence in Chapter 2.

○ Expanding coverage on sleep including information on sleep hygiene in Chapter 3.

○ Updating dietary guidelines in Chapter 7.

○ Updating physical activity guidelines in Chapter 8.

○ Expanding the section on financial management in Chapter 9.

We are thankful to all reviewers who read and provided feedback on various editions of this workbook. We are particularly thankful to reviewers of the fifth edition, including Jolynn Gardner, University of St. Thomas; Karen M. Hunter, Eastern Kentucky University; Adam Knowlden, University of Cincinnati; and Kristin Nesvacil, Illinois State University, all of whom gave specific feedback in preparation of the sixth edition. Finally, we are thankful to the students enrolled in our courses, Stress Management, Stress and Health, and Stress Reduction. Our students have been sources of great inspiration for us. They have provided valuable contributions to the organization, content, and usefulness of the material presented in the workbook. At the same time, they have incorporated these techniques in their lives and provided us with "hands-on" evidence about the utility and meaningfulness of these techniques.

John A. Romas
Manoj Sharma
Fall 2012

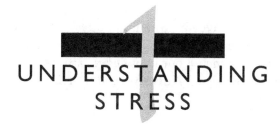

UNDERSTANDING STRESS

STRESS MANAGEMENT PRINCIPLE

" It is not the stressor but your perception of the stress that is important. "

Please complete the pre-course assessment in the Personal Assessment Log at the beginning of the workbook or online at www.pearsonhighered.com/romas.

what is stress?

If asked whether we have experienced stress in our lives, it is quite likely most of us would respond affirmatively. However, if asked to define stress, we may not be able to find appropriate words to express ourselves. Our responses might include words such as

- Pressure
- Being down
- Anger
- Anxiety
- Nervousness
- Having butterflies in the stomach
- Strain
- Negative stimulation
- Being uptight
- Depressed
- Being under the weather

○ Tension

○ Being upset

It is certainly true that these terms convey a meaning of stress. However, to comprehend stress completely, we need to explore the meaning of stress in depth. Before we proceed any further, review your knowledge, attitudes, and coping skills pertaining to stress with the help of **Worksheets 1.1, 1.2,** and **1.3** (pages 16, 17, and 18 respectively).

contemporary concepts of stress in the west

According to *Webster's New World Dictionary of American English* (2000, 4th ed.), the word *stress* is derived from the Latin word *strictus,* meaning "hardship, adversity, or affliction." It later evolved as *estresse* in Old French and *stresse* in Middle English. This word has been used in the physical sciences, medical sciences, psychology, and behavioral sciences. **Stress** has been defined from three perspectives—namely, as environmental or *external* to the body, as a mental or *internal* state of tension, and as the body's own *physical* reaction (Rice, 1999). We present the concept of stress as it has evolved in the West from response-based to event-based, and then to the interactional model. These models help explain the complex phenomenology of stress.

RESPONSE-BASED CONCEPT OF STRESS

In the Western world, the first attempts at defining stress in a psychological and behavioral context originated with the work of physiologist Walter Cannon, who defined stress as a "fight or flight" syndrome; that is, when an organism is stressed, it responds either by fighting with the **stressor** or by running away from it (Cannon, 1932). This concept gained further understanding with the work of Hans Selye on the *general adaptation syndrome* (Selye, 1936, 1974a, 1974b, 1982). While attempting to isolate a new sex hormone in rats, he observed that when injected with ovarian extracts, their adrenal glands (endocrine glands located over the kidneys that pour their secretions directly into the bloodstream) secreted corticoid hormones (a steroid), their thymus and lymph nodes became smaller in size, and they developed stomach ulcers. Later, he found that disparate events like cold, heat, infection, injury, loss of blood, and pain also produced similar responses. He labeled this gamut of responses as the general adaptation syndrome (GAS), composed of the following three stages (Figure 1.1, page 3):

○ **Stage 1: Alarm Reaction** In the alarm reaction phase, the organism's homeostasis, or balance, is disrupted. The endocrine glands become active—particularly the adrenal glands that secrete corticosteroid, which supply a ready source of energy to the body. This is accompanied by a shrinkage of lymphatic structures, decrease in blood volume, and ulcers in the stomach.

○ **Stage 2: Stage of Resistance** The stage of resistance occurs with continued exposure to the "agent" that elicited the response. In this stage, alarm reaction changes cease and opposite changes occur, such as increase in blood volume. The adaptation energy continues to deplete.

○ **Stage 3: Exhaustion** Exhaustion causes permanent damage to the system. If the agent is not removed, the organism's energy depletes and death may ensue.

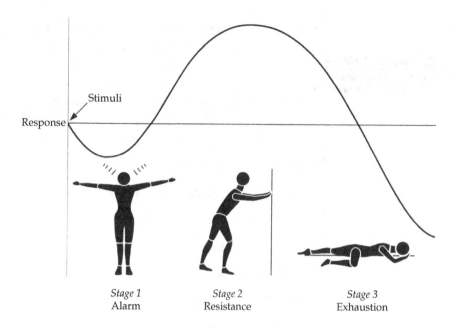

Figure 1.1 Stages of Selye's General Adaptation Syndrome

On this basis, Selye defined stress as "a nonspecific response of the body to any demand made upon it" (Selye, 1936, 1974a, 1974b, 1982). Selye, in his later work, found that the same arousal response can be evoked by different situations. Situations that are productive to the organism were labeled as *eustress*; others that are harmful were labeled as *distress* (Selye, 1982). This model of stress was response-based and physiological in its orientation. Many Russian scientists (such as Boris Aleshin, Igor Eskin, Vassily Komissarenko, etc.) also tested the model and found it to be useful (Viru, 2002). However, the main criticism leveled at this conceptualization has been its neglect of the situational and individual contexts in which stress occurs (Genest & Genest, 1987).

EVENT-BASED CONCEPT OF STRESS

The early work of Thomas Holmes and Richard Rahe (1967) focused on stressful events and constructed a Social Readjustment Rating Scale (SRRS) to assess the amount of stress to which an individual is exposed. The scale Holmes and Rahe developed assesses stress by applying weighted life change units to events in a person's life. These weights are based upon the estimated amount of change or readjustment required for each event on the part of the individual experiencing it. Estimates of this scale have been derived from ratings obtained from a sample of primarily white, middle-class adults. The total life stress experienced during a period of time is assessed by summing the weights, or life change units, of the 43 events represented on the SRRS. Before you proceed any further, complete **Worksheet 1.4** (page 20), keeping in mind the events that you have experienced during the past year.

During the 1970s the life events concept was very popular. Holmes (1979) estimated that as many as 1,000 publications appeared based on SRRS during the 1970s. Some other scales were also developed based on this concept—including, the Recent Life Changes Questionnaire (RLCQ) (Rahe, 1974) and the PERI Life Events Scale (Dohrenwend, Krasnoff, Askenasy, & Dohrenwend, 1978). Based upon this concept, stressors have been defined as life events or changes that produce or have the potential to produce changes within the individual, his or her family, and his or her

Murphy's laws are popular maxims in Western culture. There are several versions of these laws available. Accounts differ as to the precise origin of these laws. It is claimed that these laws were born at Edwards Air Force Base, California, in 1949 and were named after Edward Murphy, an engineer working on Air Force Project MX981. The project was designed to see how much sudden deceleration a person can withstand in a crash (Spark, 2006). The beauty of these laws is that they provide an interesting perspective on whatever stressful situation we are experiencing. To experience a new perspective to your stressors, reflect on this list of a few of Murphy's laws.

- Nothing is as easy as it looks.

- Everything takes longer than you think.

- If anything can go wrong, it will.

- A day without a crisis is a total loss.

- Inside every large problem is a series of small problems struggling to get out.

- The other line always moves faster.

- Whatever hits the fan will not be evenly distributed.

- No matter how long or hard you shop for an item, after you have bought it, it will be on sale somewhere cheaper.

- Any tool dropped while repairing a car will roll underneath to the exact center.

- You will remember that you forgot to take out the trash when the garbage truck is two doors away.

- Friends come and go, but enemies accumulate.

- The light at the end of the tunnel is the headlamp of an oncoming train.

- The chance of the bread falling with the peanut-butter-and-jelly side down is directly proportional to the cost of the carpet.

- The repair man will never have seen a model quite like yours before.

- Beauty is only skin deep, but ugliness goes clear to the bone.

Note: Adapted from *Murphy's laws* popular in common management parlance.

surroundings. However, later work has challenged this viewpoint. It has been found that stress reactions differ as a function of (1) neurophysiological levels of response, (2) qualities of the stressor, and (3) differences among individuals (Genest & Genest, 1987). In recent years the SRRS has been used as a suicide risk scale (Blasco-Fontecilla et al., 2012) and to assess stressors in binge eating (Woods, Racine & Klump, 2010) and depressive conditions (Vaaler, Morken, Iversen, Kondziella, & Linaker, 2010). See Thoughts for Reflection 1.1, Murphy's Laws (above).

INTERACTIONAL MODEL OF STRESS

According to the interactional model of stress, which is largely accepted now, the *perception* of the stressor by the individual is the most important factor. The degree to which anyone is stressed is influenced by a variety of factors. Richard Lazarus (1966, 1984) identified four stages in the process of stress development. The first stage is the *primary appraisal* of the event. In this stage, based upon previous experiences, knowledge about oneself and knowledge about the event determine the degree of stress. If the stressor is perceived to be threatening or has caused harm or loss, then the second stage, *secondary appraisal,* takes place. If, on the other hand, the event is judged to be irrelevant or poses no threat, then stress does not develop any further. The secondary appraisal essentially constitutes how much control one has over the situation. Based upon this understanding, the individual ascertains what means of control are available to him or her. This is the third stage known as *coping.* Finally, the fourth stage, *reappraisal,* occurs, as to whether the original stressor has been effectively negated or not. Note Box 1.1, Ancient Concepts of Stress in India.

stressors

An important aspect of enhancing our understanding of stress is understanding more about *stressors.* Stressors, in a psychosocial context, are the demands from the internal or external environment that we perceive as harmful or threatening (Lazarus & Folkman, 1984). These are generally divided into two general classes: discrete, major, stressful **life events** and ongoing, everyday **chronic stressors** (McLean & Link, 1994).

LIFE EVENTS OR LIFE CHANGE EVENTS

Wheaton (1994, page 78) describes a life change event as a "discrete, observable, and (it is thought) an objectively reportable event that requires some social and/or psychological adjustment on part of the individual." McLean and Link (1994) have further separated life events into recent stressors (experiences occurring within the past year) and remote stressors (childhood events such as physical abuse, sexual abuse, and neglect, as well as other events that occurred before the past year). This categorization of stressors is the same categorization that we saw in the discussion of the event-based conceptualization of stress in the preceding section.

CHRONIC STRESSORS

Recent research has shown that another category of stressors is more important and prevalent than discrete life events. Since these stressors occur on a daily basis, they assume greater importance in our lives. These are labeled chronic stressors. Chronic stressors do not necessarily start as distinct events but develop as continuing problematic conditions, have a longer course of duration, and do not end with a self-limiting resolution (Wheaton, 1994). McLean and Link (1994) have classified chronic stressors into five types.

The first type consists of *persistent life difficulties* that are perceived to be of long duration and are associated with life events. However, the temporal relationships (time sequence) between persistent life difficulties and life events are "often complicated to untangle" (McLean and Link, 1994, p. 24). Examples of these include any event that requires a prolonged period of adjustment, such as a teenage son or daughter leaving home or an accident that leaves a family member disabled. The second type of chronic stressors is *role strains* that result from strain within specific roles (such as working, being in a relationship, parenting, taking care of a loved one with a serious ailment, being the breadwinner of the family) and from fulfilling multiple roles at the same time. The third category is *chronic strains* that occur from

BOX 1.1

Ancient Concepts of Stress in India

One ancient civilization that flourished around the Indus Valley and later developed into a civilization in South Asia is the country known as India. We focus on the concepts drawn from Indian culture and tradition to represent the concept of stress in the East.

The four **Vedas—Rig, Sama, Yajur,** and **Atharva**—contain over a hundred thousand verses of ancient seers and sages and form the basis of the philosophy of the East. They are supported by the *Upanishads*—108 of which have been preserved. Then there are the 18 *Puranas,* including *Srimad Bhagvatam,* the *Brahma Sutras,* which contain Vedic philosophy in the form of aphorisms, *Yogasutras* of Patanjali, *Tantaras* dealing with esoteric aspects of the spiritual quest, *Manusmriti* containing the codes of conduct, and *Bhagvad Gita,* the gist of *Vedas* (Singh, 1983). In addition, the *Charaka Samhita* and *Susruta Samhita* are the texts of the *Ayurvedic* (Indian) system of medicine.

Stress is depicted by use of terms such as *dukha* (meaning pain, misery, or suffering), *klesa* (afflictions), *kama* or *trisna* (desires), *atman* and *ahankara* (self and ego), *adhi* (mental aberrations), and *prajanparadha* (failure or lapse of consciousness) (Pestonjee, 1992). These varied depictions indicate the holistic dimension of stress in Eastern thought. Pestonjee (1992) notes that according to the *Samkhya-yoga* system the cause of stress is *avidya* or faulty reality testing of either or all of the following:

▨ *Asmita:* self-appraisal, or how one views the abilities of one's body or mind

▨ *Raga:* object appraisal, or how attached a person is to his or her materials

▨ *Dvesha:* threat appraisal, or how much a person dislikes negative happenings

▨ *Abhnivesha:* coping orientation, or nonspecific sequential response to any threat

According to the Eastern viewpoint, life situations leading to stress can be one of three kinds:

1. *Adhyatmik* (personal), consisting of pathological diseases or psychological afflictions such as jealousy, fear, anger, lust, hatred, greed, grandiosity, and depression;

2. *Adhibhotik* (situational), consisting of conflicts, competition, aggression, acts of war, and so on;

3. *Adhidevik* (environmental), due to natural calamities such as earthquakes, extremes of temperature, eruption of volcanoes, and so on;

Stress operates through **four levels of stressors:**

1. **Prosupta** (dormant stressors): Any mental process is potentially stressful and can become stressful just as any seed has the potential to germinate into a plant. For example, a student might imagine that he is going to be severely reprimanded if he is late for class. This imagination would be a dormant stressor.

2. **Tonu** (tenuous or weak stressors): These are stressors of insufficient intensity and urgency that are kept in check by more powerful stressors. For example, when one is hungry, the hunger response (powerful stressor) would override worrying about being late for class (tenuous or weak stressor).

3. **Vichchinna** (intercepted stressors): These stressors alternate between stages of dormancy and manifestation. For example, a student who is reprimanded for coming late to class subsequently tries to come on time. The student has a stressor that will manifest when she becomes late. This is an intercepted stressor.

4. **Udara** (operative stressors): These stressors have found complete expression in behavior. For example, a student who has conditioned his behavior to be on time for class is exhibiting this behavior because of an operative stressor.

Hence, Eastern thought primarily places emphasis on the powers of the individual in coping with stress.

(continued)

BOX 1•1

Ancient Concepts of Stress in India

The individual can, with the help of *vidya* or *gyana* (knowledge and correct perception), understand the situation correctly, with adequate practice (*sadhana*) apply appropriate skills to reduce undue response to stressors, and ultimately develop a wholesome attitude devoid of manifest stress (*samadhi bhavana*). This is a simple explanation of the Eastern concept of stress that places an emphasis on the "correct perception" of any event by an individual in dealing with stress.

Note: Listing of pronunciation of foreign words is provided on page 233.

the response of one social group to another. Examples of these include the result of overt and covert, intentional and unintentional discriminatory behaviors due to race, ethnicity, class, gender, sexual orientation, or disability. The fourth category of chronic stressors consists of *community-wide strains,* or stressors that operate at an ecological level, such as residing in a high-crime area. The fifth category is *daily hassles,* such as waiting too long in a line or being stuck in traffic.

ANOTHER TYPE OF STRESSOR: THE NONEVENT

Besides acute life events and chronic stressors, the research literature also describes nonevents as stressors. Nonevents have been defined as desired or anticipated events that do not occur as desirable events, or do not occur even though their occurrence is normative for people of a certain group (Wheaton, 1994).

effects of stress on the body

Another aspect of understanding the concept of stress is the effect that stress has on the body. Visualizing these abstract concepts in the form of models is generally a helpful approach to enhance our understanding. Figure 1.2 (page 8) attempts to present these concepts in a model that is generally well accepted.

Various *life situations* from the internal or external environment—including loss, change, sickness, acute life events, and chronic stressors—might contribute to problematic relationships and poor financial management that affect us. These stressors are *perceived* by the cerebral cortex, the part of the brain responsible for judgment, decision making, and other higher functions. This interpretation is modified based upon our personalities, behavioral styles, values, beliefs, norms, and attitudes. Before we proceed any further, identify your personality type with the help of **Worksheet 1.5** (page 23).

The way we behave day to day constitutes our behavioral style. This topic is discussed in greater detail in Chapter 4. After perception, the next stage in the development of stress is the *emotional arousal* that triggers activity in the limbic system. The limbic system is the primitive part of the brain that is the seat of various emotions such as anger, fear, insecurity, and worry. Emotional arousal activates the *physiological response,* which is manifested by stimulation of the endocrine glands and the autonomic nervous system. The **endocrine glands** pour their secretions directly into the bloodstream. These secretions are called **hormones**. Hormones are essential chemicals that have a wide range of effects on the body. They need to be produced in optimum amounts in order for the body

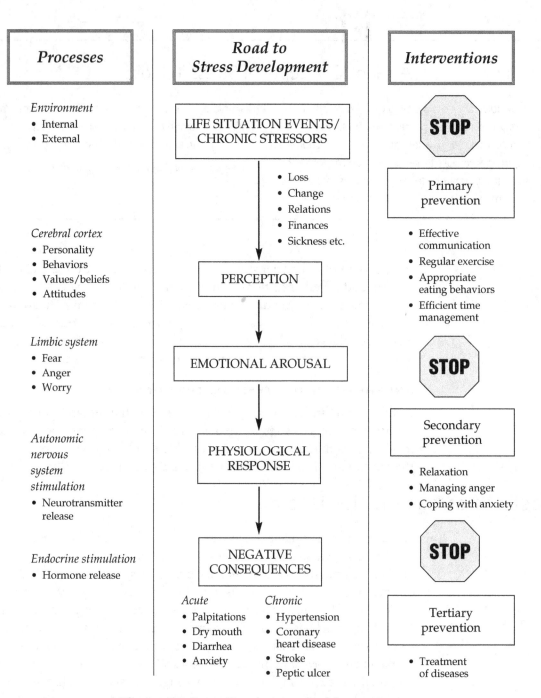

Figure 1.2 Stress Development and Intervention

to function normally. An excess or lack of these vital substances can lead to a variety of pathological (disease-related) disorders. The *autonomic nervous system* is the part of the central nervous system (brain and spinal cord) that regulates the functioning of vital organs. It consists of the sympathetic and the parasympathetic nervous systems. In simplistic terms it can be said that the sympathetic nervous system is responsible for spending energy, and the parasympathetic nervous system is responsible for conserving energy in the body. Figure 1.3 (page 9) depicts the complex physiological changes that take place in the body as a result of stress.

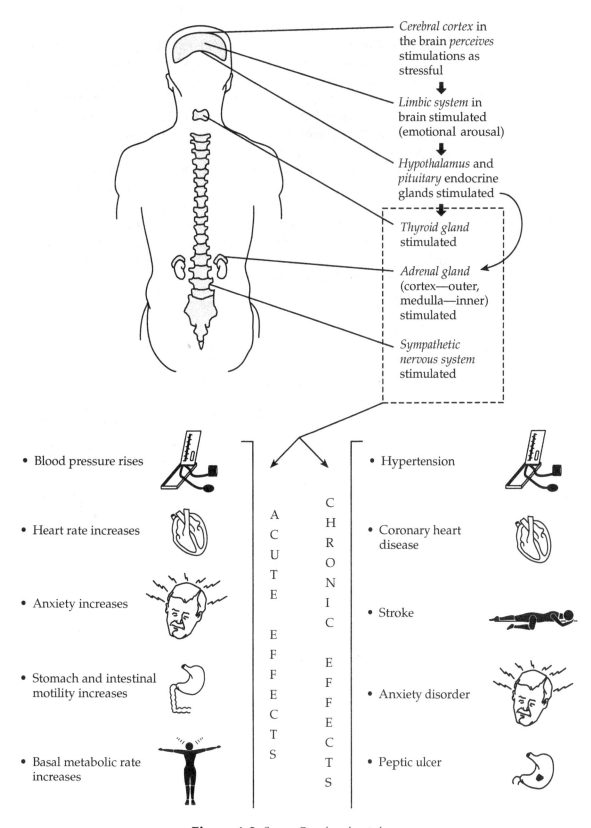

Figure 1.3 Stress Psychophysiology

The net result of these physiological activities (endocrine and autonomic nervous system stimulation) is the production of a variety of chemicals in the body (Andrews & Neises, 2012; Nejtek, 2002; Nicolaids, 2002). More often than not these chemical by-products do not get used and accumulate within the body. These chemical by-products are responsible for the *negative consequences* in the body. Stress produces both acute, or short-term, immediate effects, and chronic, or long-term effects. Figure 1.4 (below) presents the various immediate signs and symptoms of acute stress on the human body.

Stress, because of its chronic effects, can be a direct causative factor, an indirect contributory factor, a precipitating factor, or an aggravating factor for various diseases. Some of the pathological signs, symptoms, and diseases commonly associated with stress are anxiety disorders, insomnia, hypertension, stroke, coronary heart disease, ulcers, migraine headaches, tension headaches, rheumatoid arthritis, temporomandibular joint syndrome, bronchial asthma, and backache (Greenberg, 2010; Rice, 1999).

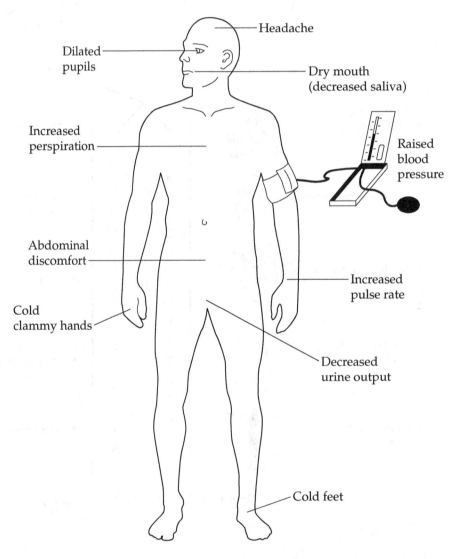

Figure 1.4 Physiological Signs and Symptoms of Acute Stress on the Body

stress in the overall context

We have discussed the concept of stress from an Eastern and Western perspective, how it has developed over time, and the effects of stress on the human body. This discussion has been medical, physiological, philosophical, and behavioral in its connotation. What is also required in this conceptualization is the historical, sociocultural, political, and organizational context in which we experience stress.

From time immemorial, human life has been ridden with stress. In premodern times there were greater threats from natural calamities, extremes of temperature, pestilence, and so on. In modern times, although industrialization has provided many facilities and improvements in the physical quality of life for many of us, these stressors have been replaced by a faster pace of life, rapidly changing technology, divergence in morality, increasing social complexity, and so on. The student, the worker, the executive, and all other people today have to face greater stress than their counterparts of yesteryear. Woolfolk and Lehrer (1993) note that present society has become individualistic and materialistic in contrast to the communal and spiritual society of the past. Never before has a large percentage of the population been without durable and dependable social support in its proper and adequate form. This lack of support is indeed a great source of stress.

In the organizational context, which could be a work setting, school setting, and/or community setting, stress has been studied quite extensively. Beer and Newman (1978) have defined job stress in terms of interaction of the person with job-related factors that disrupt or enhance his or her psychological and physiological condition. This organizational stress is further heightened for people in certain situations, such as women who have to accomplish multiple roles and students who are constantly in a phase of transition. In addition, the crisis of the modern human also lies in finding meaning to his or her activities. Often we are unable to link meaning and importance to what we are doing in daily life. In the absence of these meaningful activities with coherence and lawfulness, stress manifestations increase (Antonovsky, 1987; Shepperd & Kashani, 1991). Furthermore, despite all advancements, for a vast majority of people, primarily in the third world, basic stress is still tied into making two ends meet and mustering enough for food, clothing, and shelter. Therefore, understanding historical, sociocultural, political, and organizational factors in our lives is essential for dealing with and managing stress more effectively. Thoughts for Reflection 1.2, Why Stress Exists (page 12), will help you reflect upon some of the factors affecting modern life.

A comprehensive stress management program needs to address all these contexts and perspectives in order for the program to be successful. It will be our attempt in this workbook to try to do justice in this regard.

Another point that needs to be emphasized is that stress management is essentially a preventive approach. In preventive medicine, prevention occurs at three levels: primary, secondary, and tertiary. *Primary prevention* is the level where the intervention occurs before the disease. In stress management, it is the level regarding "perception" of the stressor. *Secondary prevention* is the level of intervention when the disease process has started. In stress management, it is the stage when emotional arousal and physiological activation have occurred. *Tertiary prevention* is the level when disease has already caused damage. In stress management, it is the stage when negative consequences have set in and then we intervene. It is akin to stamping out the fire after the inferno has engulfed the property. In this context it is worth noting that some experts view stress as a risk factor; therefore, stress

Present-day life is more complex than ever before. A reflection on some of the factors responsible for this complexity will help you cope with stress better. Stress affects our personal, academic, family, and work lives. Following is a list of some of these factors:

Intricacy of Social Fabric. In our personal, academic, and work lives, we have come to a point where our relationships have become extremely complex and challenging. Much of our life revolves around getting into, being in, and getting out of relationships. All these events are potentially stressful.

Divergence in Morality and Ethics. We have developed a value system that presents us with highly divergent and conflicting standpoints on various life issues such as terrorism, war, and ecological concerns. Adjustments and responses to these contradictions are stressful.

Conflicting Expectations. Most of the time, in our academic or work life as well as our personal life, we do not know what is expected of us. This unclarity about our role is a stressful factor.

Marginal Communication. Poor and ineffective communication in our day-to-day life is a major source of discomfort and stress.

Rapid Change in Technology. The advancement in science and technology has pervaded all walks of life. Inherent in this change is stress.

Lack of Proper Training to Do What One Is Being Asked to Do. In our work life, owing to the gap between "education" and "profession," we are at times unable to do what is being asked of us. This gap is a strong source of stress.

Ineffective Management Systems. Despite the innovation and implementation of a wide variety of management systems that have enhanced production and have been responsible for quality products, we have been unable to develop a management system that completely rids us of stress.

Lack of Job Security. In present times, we do not know if we will be able to remain in our job or not. This insecurity provides ample stress in life.

Limited or No Organizational Loyalty. These days many of us cannot associate ourselves with the job that we perform and the organization with which we work. This is an extremely stressful factor.

Economic Overextension. Pressure that money exerts in all walks of life is a potent stressor.

management, according to them, is primary prevention. However, we would like to view stress as a disease in its developmental form and have, therefore, classified stress management with the various levels of prevention described previously.

Finally, the importance of one's *perception and attitude* in comprehending stress and dealing with it cannot be overemphasized. Thoughts for Reflection 1.3, On Attitude (page 13) reinforces our belief in the importance of developing a *positive attitude,* which is at the core of all stress management efforts. Positive mental attitude is also discussed in many martial arts. The Stress Management Principle at the beginning of this chapter is also in line with this ideology. It is hoped that the reader will not only memorize this principle, but also try to incorporate it in his or her life.

■ Attitude determines our behavior.

■ It is up to each one of us to choose how we will respond to any situation.

■ What happens to us in life has relatively little effect compared to how we choose to respond. If you *choose* to get upset, worked up, and worried, even a small, trivial event, colored with your imagination, may appear to be devastating. However, if you *choose* to envision the situation in perspective, and not get upset or worried, then your coping skills are enhanced.

■ Effort and directed determination are required for changing attitude.

■ Understanding the importance of *attitude* and its impact upon behavior is more significant than being factual, scientific, and analytical.

CHAPTER REVIEW

summary points

○ Walter Cannon defined stress as a "fight or flight" syndrome; that is, when an organism is stressed it either responds by fighting with the stressor or by running away from it.

○ Hans Selye described the *general adaptation syndrome,* consisting of *alarm reaction, stage of resistance,* and *exhaustion.* On this basis he defined stress as the "nonspecific response of the body to any demand made upon it."

○ Thomas Holmes and Richard Rahe constructed the Social Readjustment Rating Scale (SRRS) to assess the amount of stress experienced by an individual as a result of changing life events.

○ Richard Lazarus described stress development in *four stages—primary appraisal, secondary appraisal, coping,* and *reappraisal.*

○ Stressors are of two types: (1) acute life events and (2) chronic stressors.

○ Acute life events are of two types: (1) recent (within one year) and (2) remote (beyond one year).

○ Chronic stressors are of five types: (1) persistent life difficulties, (2) role strains, (3) chronic strains, (4) community-wide strains, and (5) daily hassles.

○ Nonevents have also been defined as stressful because of perceived expectations.

○ According to Eastern thought, stress is described as *dukha* (pain, misery, suffering), *klesa* (afflictions), *kama* or *trisna* (desires), *atman* and *ahankara* (self and ego), *adhi* (mental aberrations), and *prajanparadha* (failure or lapse of consciousness). The main cause is *avidya* (faulty reality testing).

- Type A personality people (characterized by hurrying nature, competitive zeal, dominating nature, and fast pace of life) are more prone to stress. Hardiness is exhibited by individuals with control, commitment, and challenge.

- A generally accepted model of stress development consists of life situations that are perceived as stressful and that lead to an emotional and physiological response, thus leading to negative consequences.

- The physiological response in stress is composed of endocrine stimulation and sympathetic nervous system overactivity.

- Some pathological signs, symptoms, and diseases associated with stress are anxiety disorders, insomnia, hypertension, stroke, coronary heart disease, ulcers, migraine headaches, tension headaches, rheumatoid arthritis, temporomandibular joint syndrome, bronchial asthma, and backache.

- Stress, besides medical, psychological, behavioral, and philosophical contexts, also needs to be understood in sociocultural, political, and organizational perspectives in order to devise a meaningful stress management effort.

important terms defined

chronic stressors: A distinct subgroup of stressors (environmental events) that are ongoing and everyday issues affecting or having the potential to influence a person's body, mind, family, or community—for example, driving every day during the rush hour in high traffic for school. *See also* **life events, stressors.**

endocrine glands: Organs in the body that pour their secretions (hormones) directly into the bloodstream. These are also known as ductless glands. Examples of these glands include the pituitary gland located near the center of the brain, thyroid and parathyroid glands located in the neck region, islet cells of Langerhans in the pancreas gland located in the abdominal region, cortex of the adrenal (suprarenal) glands located on the top of the kidneys, testes in males, and ovaries in females. *See also* **hormones.**

hormones: These are secretions from the endocrine glands—for example, thyroxin hormone from the thyroid gland, adrenocorticotropic hormone (ACTH) from the pituitary gland, insulin from the pancreas, or testosterone from the testes.

life events: A distinct subgroup of stressors (environmental events) that are discrete, major happenings affecting or having the potential to influence one's body, mind, family, or community—for example, a death in the family. *See also* **chronic stressors, stressors.**

stress: The response of the body, mind, and behaviors as a result of encountering stressors (external events), interpreting these, making judgments about controlling or influencing the outcomes of these events.

stressors: The various external events that pose an actual or perceived threat to the body or mind.

websites to explore

AMERICAN INSTITUTE OF STRESS

www.stress.org/

The website provides information about the American Institute of Stress, a nonprofit organization established in 1978 to serve as a clearinghouse for information on all stress-related subjects. Among the founding members were Hans Selye, Linus Pauling, Alvin Toffler, Bob Hope, Michael DeBakey, Herbert Benson, and Ray Rosenman. The institute provides membership and fellowships to prominent physicians, health professionals, and individuals interested in exploring the effects of stress on health and quality of life. The authors of this book are fellows of this Institute.

▨ Use this website to explore the contributions of some of the noted personalities in the stress field. Also check out the monthly newsletter of the organization.

INTERNATIONAL STRESS MANAGEMENT ASSOCIATION

www.isma.org.uk/

The website provides information about the United Kingdom–based charitable organization International Stress Management Association. The association has a multidisciplinary professional membership. It has been established to promote scientific knowledge and best practices in the prevention and reduction of human stress. It started as an offshoot of the American Association for the Advancement of Tension Control in 1974 and was formally formed under the present name in 1989. It has branches in 12 countries.

▨ Using the website, explore the recent conferences and other events related to stress. Which one would you like to participate in, and why? Can you also get more web-based information on the chosen event and have virtual participation if not real?

INTERNATIONAL ORGANIZATION OF PSYCHOPHYSIOLOGY

http://iopworld.org

This is the official website of the International Organization of Psychophysiology. Formed in 1982, this organization has affiliation with the United Nations and publishes the International Journal of Psychophysiology. *It maintains relations with over 2,000 organizations and has membership from close to 50 nations. It organizes the Annual World Congress of Psychophysiology.*

▨ Explore the website to find information about the Century Award that this organization presented to eminent psychophysiologists. Can you identify the contributions of any one of these leaders?

JOURNAL OF PSYCHOPHYSIOLOGY

www.hogrefe.com/periodicals/journal-of-psychophysiology/

This is the website of an international journal that is an official publication of the Federation of European Psychophysiological Societies. *The journal presents original research in all fields employing psychophysiological techniques. The disciplines include psychology, physiology, clinical psychology, psychiatry, neurosciences, pharmacology, and genetics. The journal also includes contributions from animal research and new methodologies, such as recording technology, data reduction, statistical methods, as well as computer hardware and software.*

▨ Explore the current abstracts from the recent issues on the website and use your library to locate and read any one article of your interest.

What Do You Know About Stress?

We all have some knowledge about stress. However, much of what we know about stress is based on intuition, opinions, beliefs, biases, hunches, and misinformation. These questions will provide you with some feedback regarding what you know about stress. Read each statement and mark T (true) or F (false).

_____ 1. One major stressful event such as the death of someone close causes many more ill effects of stress than small, everyday hassles.

_____ 2. Stressors will always precipitate stress.

_____ 3. Stress decreases the amount of saliva in the mouth, resulting in a feeling of "cotton mouth."

_____ 4. Energy is conserved during stress.

_____ 5. People who are not competitive and have no time urgency have more stress.

_____ 6. A person who often says "no" loses many friends, which results in stress.

_____ 7. Drinking coffee or tea reduces stress.

_____ 8. The good thing about smoking is that it relaxes the body and relieves stress.

_____ 9. Exercise helps to build the body but robs it of vital energy, causing stress.

_____ 10. Acquired behaviors for stress cannot be changed.

FEEDBACK ON WORKSHEET 1.1

1. F Research shows that everyday hassles are even more detrimental to one's health than major life changes (Lazarus, 1984; Monroe & McQuaid, 1994).

2. F Stressors only have the *potential* of eliciting stress. How we react is most important (Greenberg, 2008; J. C. Smith, 1993).

3. T Stress leads to two basic physiological processes—stimulation of the autonomic nervous system and the endocrine system. One of the manifestations of these physiological effects is dry mouth (Guyton & Hall, 2006).

4. F During stress the sympathetic nervous system is activated, resulting in expenditure of energy (Greenberg, 2008; Selye, 1936).

5. F People characterized by excessive competitive drive, aggressiveness, impatience, and a hurried sense of time urgency (Type A) are more prone to stress than people with Type B personality traits characterized by no free-floating hostility, no time urgency, and little competitive spirit (Friedman & Rosenman, 1959).

6. F Saying no—expressing oneself and satisfying one's own needs while not hurting others—is assertiveness and helps to reduce stress (Bower & Bower, 1976; Fensterheim & Fensterheim, 1975; M. J. Smith, 1975).

7. F Colas, coffee, tea, and chocolate contain caffeine, which is a pseudostressor or a sympathomimetic drug that causes a stresslike reaction (Girdano, Everly, & Dusek, 2012; Greenberg, 2010).

8. F Nicotine, found in tobacco, is also a sympathomimetic agent (Greenberg, 2010).

9. F Exercise is good not only for physical health but also for psychological well-being (U.S. Department of Health and Human Services [USDHHS], 1996).

10. F The basis for stress management programs is that by reducing stressful behaviors and increasing healthful behaviors, one can better manage stress in life (Enelow & Henderson, 1975; Green & Kreuter, 2004; Kasl & Cobb, 1966).

How Are Your Stress Coping Skills?

We all cope with stress in our lives. However, some of us are overwhelmed by it. Likewise, some situations trigger more stress than others. The following ten statements are designed to provide you with some feedback regarding your coping skills concerning stress. Please read each statement and rate your skill.

Item	Excellent	Very Good	Satis-factory	Needs Improvement	Needs A lot of Improvement
1. Ability to relax whenever I want to relax					
2. Ability to assert myself while communicating					
3. Ability to keep my anger under control					
4. Ability to resolve my conflicts at work and home					
5. Ability to manage my time efficiently					
6. Ability to exercise regularly					
7. Ability to cope with my anxiety over *future* events					
8. Ability to cope with my anxiety over *past* events					
9. Ability to balance my healthy eating behaviors					
10. Ability to set and implement realistic goals in order to accomplish desired objectives in life					

FEEDBACK ON WORKSHEET 1.2

This worksheet enhances your own understanding of the various coping skills that you possess with respect to managing stress. The areas in which you do not have adequate skills can be acquired with patience and practice. The chapters in this workbook will help you identify skills that you need to develop further.

What Kind of Attitude Do You Have About Stress?

All of us perceive stress differently and have different attitudes about stress. Some attitudes are helpful in coping with stress, but others are not so helpful. The following ten statements are designed to provide you with some feedback regarding your attitudes about stress. Read each of the following statements and rate your agreement or disagreement with the statements.

Item	Strongly Agree	Agree	Disagree	Strongly Disagree	No Opinion
1. People with stress are weak-minded.					
2. Stress management programs do not work.					
3. Stress management programs help people.					
4. Stress cannot be managed.					
5. There is no such thing as "stress."					
6. Other people cause my stress.					
7. I never experience stress, but other people around me are stressed.					
8. Stress is not harmful.					
9. The more we worry about future events, the better we can shape them.					
10. Setting a goal, making a plan, and implementing the plan can reduce one's stress levels.					

FEEDBACK ON WORKSHEET 1.3

1. All of us experience stress from time to time; it is not a question of being weak-minded or not.

2–4. Evidence indicates that stress management programs are successful in reducing the levels of stress that we experience in our lives. These programs substantially reduce stress and the harmful consequences associated with stress.

5. Scientific research demonstrates that all of us experience stress from time to time; the only difference is how we choose to respond to it. Denial leads us nowhere. Prudence lies in accepting reality and finding the most appropriate way to deal with stress in our lives.

6. No other person can disturb our peace of mind if we choose not to be disturbed. Therefore, only we are responsible for our stress.

7. We have to be careful not to project our stress upon others. All of us encounter stress in our lives.

8. Stress has been known to be associated (directly and indirectly) with a variety of disorders, such as hypertension, coronary heart disease, stroke, headaches, and bronchial asthma (Greenberg, 2008). Denying that stress is harmful is a negative attitude that hinders our learning about the basics of stress management.

9. Worrying about the future only adds to our stress and is of no use.

10. Scientific evidence indicates that setting a goal and implementing a plan to achieve it is an effective way to reduce stress.

The Social Readjustment Rating Scale (SRRS)

Focus on the events that you have experienced in the past year. For the events experienced, enter the mean value in the score column.

Rank	Life Event	Mean Value	Score
1	Death of spouse/significant other	100	_____
2	Divorce	73	_____
3	Marital separation	65	_____
4	Jail term	63	_____
5	Death of a close family member	63	_____
6	Personal injury or illness	53	_____
7	Marriage/new life partner	50	_____
8	Fired at work	47	_____
9	Marital reconciliation	45	_____
10	Retirement	45	_____
11	Change in health of a family member	44	_____
12	Pregnancy	40	_____
13	Sex difficulties	39	_____
14	Gain of a new family member	39	_____
15	Business readjustment	39	_____
16	Change in financial state	38	_____
17	Death of a close friend	37	_____
18	Change to a different line of work	36	_____
19	Change in number of arguments with spouse/significant other	35	_____
20	Mortgage over $200,000	31	_____
21	Foreclosure of mortgage or loan	30	_____
22	Change in responsibilities at work (increase or decrease)	29	_____
23	Son or daughter leaving home	29	_____
24	Trouble with in-laws	29	_____
25	Outstanding personal achievement	28	_____

The Social Readjustment Rating Scale (SRRS) (cont'd)

Rank	Life Event	Mean Value	Score
26	Spouse/mate beginning or stopping work	26	_____
27	Beginning or ending school	26	_____
28	Change in living conditions	25	_____
29	Revision of personal habits	24	_____
30	Trouble with boss/person in authority	23	_____
31	Change in work hours or conditions	20	_____
32	Change in residence	20	_____
33	Change in schools	20	_____
34	Change in recreation	19	_____
35	Change in church activities	19	_____
36	Change in social activities	18	_____
37	Mortgage or loan less than $200,000	17	_____
38	Change in sleeping habits	16	_____
39	Change in number of family get-togethers	15	_____
40	Change in eating habits	15	_____
41	Vacation	13	_____
42	Christmas	12	_____
43	Minor violations of the law	11	_____
		TOTAL	_____

Note: Adapted from "The social readjustment scale" by T. H. Holmes & R. H. Rahe, *Journal of Psychosomatic Research, 11,* copyright 1967, Elsevier Science Ltd. Reprinted with permission from Elsevier Science Ltd., Oxford, England. Some items from the original scale have been modified to make them more contemporary.

A life change unit score between 150 and 199 shows a 37 percent chance of these stressors leading to sickness in the following year; scores between 200 and 299, a 51 percent chance; and scores over 300, a 79 percent chance (Holmes & Rahe, 1967).

The SRRS represents the early work of T. H. Holmes and R. H. Rahe. It still forms the basis for psychosocial understanding of stress. Appropriate adjustments in life events can be included to meet the needs of contemporary society.

The total score on this SRRS represents the total life change units experienced by the respondent. The scale assesses stress by applying weighted life change units to the events in a person's life. These weights are based upon the estimated amount of change or readjustment required for each event on the part of the individual experiencing it. These estimates have been derived from a sample of primarily white, middle-class adults. Therefore, the levels of life change units are subject to modification depending upon social, cultural, and other demographic variables. Furthermore, some of the events, such as mortgage, etc., have changed their contemporary significance. Despite these limitations the scale gives a fair idea regarding the stress that you have experienced in the recent past. This view was very popular in the 1970s, and a lot of research substantiated this viewpoint, correlating the higher life change unit scores with illness (Holmes, 1979; Holmes & Masuda, 1974; Rahe & Arthur, 1978).

Identifying Type of Personality

Please answer Yes or No to the following questions and count the Yes responses:

1. Do you speak quickly?

2. Do you rush through daily activities?

3. Do you get impatient when things do not move at the pace that you prefer?

4. Do you typically multitask, taking on more than one task at a time?

5. Do you talk only about topics that you are interested in when having a conversation?

6. Do you feel guilty when relaxing?

7. Do you often fail to take the time to notice the things around you?

8. Do you have sense of urgency with respect to time?

9. Are you interested in possessing things?

10. Do you compete with others?

11. Do you believe that a quick pace to life is needed?

12. Do you use a lot of gestures while talking?

13. Do you measure success in terms of numbers?

Note. Based on *Type A Behavior and Your Heart* by Meyer Friedman and Ray Rosenman, 1974, New York: Fawcett Crest.

FEEDBACK ON WORKSHEET 1.5

If the total number of your yes responses is more than 7, you are likely to be Type A in your orientation. The higher your score is from 7 toward 13, the stronger is the likelihood of your being Type A. Type A personality types exhibit excessive competitive drive, are aggressive and impatient, and always have an urgency of time. The basis of this personality is believed to be a free-floating form of generalized hostility and a sense of insecurity.

If, on the contrary, you have lower scores, you are likely to be Type B in your orientation. Type B personality types do not have an urgency of time and are not competitive; instead, they tend to be cooperative and patient. These are the happy-go-lucky kind of people.

Type A personality types have been shown to be more prone to stress and its negative consequences. However, these personality-type classifications are not rigid assessments and are more *situational* in their connotation. Importantly, they can be modified.

Health authorities have now identified the concept of **hardiness** as a characteristic that has helped some people negate self-imposed stress associated with Type A behavior. Psychologically, *hardy* individuals are characterized as having *control*, *commitment*, and *challenge*. Those with a sense of control are able to accept responsibility for their behaviors and to make changes in behaviors that they discover to be debilitating. People with a sense of commitment have good self-esteem and understand their purpose in life. People with a sense of challenge see changes in life as stimulating opportunities for personal growth.

references and further readings

Andrews, J. A., & Neises, K. D. (2012). Cells, biomarkers, and post-traumatic stress disorder: Evidence for peripheral involvement in a central disease. *Journal of Neurochemistry, 120*(1), 26–36.

Antonovsky, A. (1987). The salutogenic perspective: Toward a new view of health and illness. *Advances, 4,* 47–55.

Beer, T. A., & Newman, H. E. (1978). Job stress, employee health, and organizational effectiveness: A facet analysis, model, and literature review. *Personnel Psychology, 31,* 665–699.

Blasco-Fontecilla, H., Delgado-Gomez, D., Legido-Gil, T., de Leon, J., Perez-Rodriguez, M. M., & Baca-Garcia, E. (2012). Can the Holmes-Rahe Social Readjustment Rating Scale (SRRS) be used as a suicide risk scale? An exploratory study. *Archives of Suicide Research, 16*(1),13–28.

Bower, S. A., & Bower, G. H. (1976). *Asserting yourself.* Reading, MA: Addison-Wesley.

Cannon, W. B. (1932). *The wisdom of the body.* New York: Norton.

Dohrenwend, B. S., Krasnoff, L., Askenasy, A. R., & Dohrenwend, B. P. (1978). Exemplification of a method for scaling life events: The PERI Life Events Scale. *Journal of Health and Social Behavior, 19,* 205–229.

Enelow, A. J., & Henderson, J. B. (Eds.). (1975). *Applying behavioral science to cardiovascular risk.* New York: American Heart Association.

Fensterheim, H., & Fensterheim, B. (1975). *Don't say yes when you want to say no.* New York: David McKay.

Friedman, M., & Rosenman, R. H. (1959). Association of specific overt behavior pattern with blood and cardiovascular findings: Blood clotting time, incidence of arcus senilis, and clinical coronary artery disease. *Journal of the American Medical Association, 169,* 1286–1296.

Friedman, M., & Rosenman, R. H. (1974). *Type A behavior and your heart.* New York: Fawcett Crest.

Genest, M., & Genest, S. (1987). *Psychology and health.* Champaign, IL: Research Press.

Girdano, D. A., Everly, G. S., Jr., & Dusek, D. E. (2012). *Controlling stress and tension* (9th ed.). San Francisco: Benjamin Cummings.

Green, L. W., & Kreuter, M. W. (2004). *Health promotion planning: An educational and environmental approach* (4th ed.). Boston: McGraw-Hill.

Greenberg, J. S. (2010). *Comprehensive stress management* (12th ed.). Boston: McGraw-Hill.

Guyton, A. C., & Hall, J. E. (2006). *Textbook of medical physiology* (11th ed.). Philadelphia: Saunders.

Holmes, T. H. (1979). Development and application of a quantitative measure of life change magnitude. In J. E. Barrett, R. M. Rose, & G. L. Klerman (Eds.), *Stress and mental disorder* (pp. 37–53). New York: Raven.

Holmes, T. H., & Masuda, M. (1974). Life change and illness susceptibility. In B. S. Dohrenwend & B. P. Dohrenwend (Eds.), *Stressful life events: Their nature and effects* (pp. 49–72). New York: Wiley.

Holmes, T. H., & Rahe, R. H. (1967). The social readjustment rating scale. *Journal of Psychosomatic Research, 11,* 213–218.

Kasl, S. V., & Cobb, S. (1966). Health behavior, illness behavior, and sick role behavior. *Archives of Environmental Health, 12,* 246–266.

Lazarus, R. S. (1966). *Psychological stress and the coping process.* New York: McGraw-Hill.

Lazarus, R. S. (1984). Puzzles in the study of daily hassles. *Journal of Behavioral Medicine, 7,* 375–389.

Lazarus, R. S., & Folkman, S. (1984). *Stress, appraisal, and coping.* New York: Springer.

McLean, D. E., & Link, B. G. (1994). Unraveling complexity: Strategies to refine concepts, measures, and research designs in the study of life events and mental health. In W. R. Avison & I. H. Gotlib (Eds.), *Stress and mental health: Contemporary issues and prospects for the future* (pp. 15–42). New York: Plenum Press.

Monroe, S. M., & McQuaid, J. R. (1994). Measuring life stress and assessing its impact on mental health. In W. R. Arison & I. H. Gotlib (Eds.), *Stress and mental health: Contemporary issues and prospects for the future* (pp. 43–76). New York: Plenum Press.

Nejtek, V. A. (2002). High and low emotion events influence emotional stress perceptions and are associated with salivary cortisol response changes in a consecutive stress paradigm. *Psychoneuroendocrinology 27,* 337–352.

Nicolaids, S. (2002). A hormone-based characterization and taxonomy of stress: Possible usefulness in management. *Metabolism, 51,* 31–36.

Pestonjee, D. M. (1992). *Stress and coping: The Indian experience.* Newbury Park, CA: Sage Publications.

Rahe, R. H. (1974). The pathway between subjects' recent life changes and their near future illness reports: Representative results and methodological issues. In B. S. Dohrenwend & B. P. Dohrenwend (Eds.), *Stressful life events: Their nature and effects* (pp. 73–86). New York: Wiley.

Rahe, R. H., & Arthur, R. J. (1978). Life change and illness studies: Past history and future directions. *Journal of Human Stress, 4,* 3–15.

Rice, P. L. (1999). *Stress and health* (3rd ed.). Belmont, CA: Wadsworth.

Sapolsky, R. M. (1999). *Why zebras don't get ulcers: An updated guide to stress, stress-related diseases and coping.* New York: Freeman.

Selye, H. (1936). A syndrome produced by diverse nocuous agents. *Nature, 138,* 32.

Selye, H. (1974a). *Stress without distress.* Philadelphia: Lippincott.

Selye, H. (1974b). *The stress of life.* New York: McGraw-Hill.

Selye, H. (1982). History and present status of stress concept. In L. Goldberger & S. Breznitz (Eds.), *Handbook of stress: Theoretical and clinical aspects* (pp. 7–17). New York: Free Press.

Sheppard, J. A., & Kashani, J. V. (1991). The relationship of hardiness, gender, and stress to health outcomes in adolescents. *Journal of Personality, 59,* 747–768.

Singh, K. (1983). Hinduism. In *Religions of India* (pp. 17–74). New Delhi, India: Clarion Books.

Smith, J. C. (1993). *Understanding stress and coping.* New York: Macmillan.

Smith, M. J. (1975). *When I say no, I feel guilty.* New York: Dial Press.

Spark, N. T. (2006). *A history of Murphy's law.* Los Angeles: Periscope Film.

USDHHS (U. S. Department of Health and Human Services). (1996). *Physical activity and health: A report of the Surgeon General* (p. 4). Atlanta: U.S. Department of Health and Human Services, Centers for Disease Control and Prevention, National Center for Chronic Disease Prevention and Health Promotion.

Vaaler, A. E., Morken, G., Iversen, V. C., Kondziella, D., & Linaker, O. M. (2010). Acute Unstable Depressive Syndrome (AUDS) is associated more frequently with epilepsy than major depression. *BMC Neurology, 10,* 67.

Viru, A. (2002). Early contributions of Russian stress and exercise physiologists. *Journal of Applied Physiology, 92,* 1378–1382.

Wheaton, B. (1994). Sampling the stress universe. In W. R. Avison & I. H. Gotlib (Eds.), *Stress and mental health: Contemporary issues and prospects for the future.* New York: Plenum Press.

Woods, A. M., Racine, S. E., & Klump, K. L. (2010). Examining the relationship between dietary restraint and binge eating: Differential effects of major and minor stressors. *Eating Behaviors, 11*(4), 276–280.

Woolfolk, R. L., & Lehrer, P. M. (1993). The context of stress management. In P. M. Lehrer & R. L. Woolfolk (Eds.), *Principles and practice of stress management* (2nd ed.) (pp. 3–14). New York: Guilford Press.

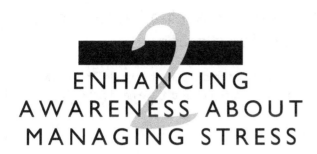

ENHANCING AWARENESS ABOUT MANAGING STRESS

awareness about managing stress

In Chapter 1 we focused on developing knowledge about stress. Although knowledge is essential for any behavior change to take place, often it is not sufficient (Bandura, 1995). Besides knowledge, what is also required for behavior change are enhanced personal awareness, appropriate attitudes, suitable beliefs, a well-developed set of skills, and germane environmental conditions (Green & Kreuter, 2005). Since the 1950s behavioral and social scientists have developed several theories and models to enhance our understanding of the complex process of behavioral change (Glanz, Rimer, & Viswanath, 2008). One such model is the health belief model, which attempts to explain and predict health behaviors in terms of certain belief patterns (Becker, 1974; Hochbaum, 1958, Sharma & Romas, 2012). Box 2.1, The Health Belief Model and Its Application to Stress Management: An In-depth Investigation (page 28), presents this model as an in-depth investigation and discusses some beliefs that you need to be aware of in order to manage and reduce stress in your personal life. Likewise, Box 2.2, Social Cognitive Theory and Its Application to Stress Management: An In-depth Investigation (page 29), presents the applications of social cognitive theory, another popular theory in health behavior (Bandura, 1995, 2004; Sharma & Romas, 2012), as an in-depth investigation.

It is evident from the health belief model that an understanding of what needs to be changed is an essential starting point for any behavior change to take place. An understanding of the potential stressors in our life (cues to action), potential negative consequences from these stressors (perceived susceptibility), and the seriousness of these negative consequences (perceived severity) is important for us to begin managing and reducing stress in our personal lives. Therefore, in this chapter we will identify the acute and chronic manifestations of stress in

BOX 2·1

The Health Belief Model and Its Application to Stress Management: An In-depth Investigation

The health belief model has several components that attempt to explain or predict behavior change. The following table presents the components of the health belief model and discusses some beliefs that we need to be aware of in order to manage and reduce stress in our personal lives.

Component	What It Means	Stress Management/ Reducing Beliefs
Perceived susceptibility	Belief that a person may acquire a disease or enter a harmful state as a result of a particular behavior	If we believe that stress has the potential to produce some *negative consequences*, then it is likely that we will act to reduce stress in our lives.
Perceived severity	Belief in the extent of harm that can result from the acquired disease or harmful state as a result of a particular behavior	If we believe that stress has the potential to produce *serious* negative consequences, such as heart disease, then we will act to reduce stress in our lives.
Perceived benefits	Belief in the benefit of the methods suggested for reducing the risk or seriousness of the disease or harmful state resulting from a particular behavior	If we believe that by learning stress management techniques, such as relaxation, we will *benefit*, then it is likely that we will follow these new behaviors.
Perceived barriers	Belief concerning actual and imagined costs of following the new behavior	If we can reassure ourselves that applying stress management techniques results in a minimal *expense* and maximal benefit in the long run, then it is likely that we will follow these new behaviors.
Cues to action	Precipitating force that makes a person feel the need to take action	If we can identify the personal stressors that *trigger* negative consequences for us, then it is likely that we will follow the new behaviors that reduce stress in our lives.
Self-efficacy	Confidence to follow a behavior	If we can *practice*, in small steps, new stress management behaviors and demonstrate that we have acquired mastery over these new behaviors, then it is likely that we will follow these new behaviors.

BOX **2·2**

Social Cognitive Theory and Its Application to Stress Management: An In-depth Investigation

The social cognitive theory is a very "robust" theory that talks about triadic reciprocality among personal determinants, environmental conditions, and learning of behavior. Although all constructs of this theory are difficult to modify in any single personal health program, the reader can choose and select some constructs from the theory to assist with behavior change(s) in his or her personal life. Selected constructs are presented in the following table.

Construct	What It Means	Stress Management/Reducing Application
Expectations	Anticipations that we have about outcomes as a result of engaging in a desired behavior	For example, if we want to start a daily relaxation routine to reduce stress, then we need to (1) reflect on all possible benefits other than just stress relief for engaging in this behavior and (2) make a complete list of potential benefits.
Expectancies	Values that we place on the anticipated outcome as a result of engaging in the chosen behavior	For example, we think of all the reasons to start relaxation and place most value on improved concentration and least value on finding the purpose of life (self-realization). We then need to constantly remind ourselves about the outcomes that we value most rather than all the outcomes. Such reminders will reinforce the performance of the behavior.
Self-efficacy	Behavior and situation-specific confidence that we have in our ability to perform a behavior	For example, to start a daily relaxation routine, we need to break the steps into manageable units, remind ourselves about people we like who use relaxation, and have friends and family who compliment us whenever they find us practicing relaxation.
Self-control	Explicit and specific goal setting for behavior change	For example, if we want to start a daily relaxation routine, we need to specify when—which date and at what time—we will start. What will be the duration of each session? What audio aid will be used? What self-reward will be given?
Situational perception	How we look at the environment and interpret it	First, we would need to check for any misperceptions and correct these. For example, you have been left by the person you love. Instead of thinking that you have been "rejected" and feeling depressed, you can focus on thinking of this as a change. Second, we need to look at the environmental event and think about the advantages and disadvantages of this situation, and then, focus on the advantages for self. The possible advantages could be fewer arguments, the possibility of starting a new relationship, and so on.

our life, discern some potential personal stressors, and recognize behaviors that need to be changed. In the subsequent chapters of this workbook we will build our confidence in practicing new behaviors that help us manage or reduce stress in our lives (self-efficacy), recognize the benefits of these behaviors (perceived benefits), and identify barriers (perceived barriers) that prevent us from applying these new behaviors.

First, from the social cognitive theory, it is evident that fear-based or negative outcomes are not as useful in changing behavior as are positive outcomes. Therefore, thinking about outcomes (**expectations**) and their value (**expectancies**) is very helpful for motivation. Second, the need to regularly practice behavior in small graded steps (**self-efficacy**) and having specific, explicit goals (**self-control**) is essential. Therefore, efforts have been made to build upon these two constructs. Finally, correct perception (**situational perception**) is very important.

acute manifestations of stress

We have already seen in Chapter 1 that stress produces a number of immediate manifestations. These include anxiety, raised blood pressure, increased heart rate, increased intestinal motility, dry mouth, cold, clammy hands, and increased perspiration. Manifestations occur soon after a stressor has affected our body. We need to identify changes in our body. Therefore, you should now complete **Worksheet 2.1** (page 36) and find out how your body reacts to acute stress.

chronic manifestations of stress

Chronic stress is also harmful to us. Chronic stress can permanently raise our blood pressure levels. This condition is known as hypertension. Hypertension has been identified as a risk factor for coronary heart disease (CHD) and cerebrovascular disease, or stroke. The cause for 90 percent of these cases of hypertension is not known, and these are labeled as essential hypertension (Labarthe & Roccella, 1993). Stress plays a substantial role in causing coronary heart disease (Kubzansky & Koenen, 2009; Hamet & Tremblay, 2002; Matthews & Gump, 2002; Von Kanel, Mills, Fainman, & Dimsdale, 2001). Figure 2.1 (page 31) shows how stress is related to hypertension and coronary heart disease.

Besides hypertension, CHD, and stroke, stress is related as a risk factor to many other physical ailments. Some of these are migraine headaches, peptic ulcers, arthritis, colitis, diarrhea, asthma, cardiac arrhythmias, sexual problems, circulatory problems (cold hands and feet), muscle tension, allergies, backache, temporomandibular joint syndrome, and cancer (Girdano, Everly, & Dusek, 2012; Greenberg, 2010; Rice, 1999; Smith, 1993). Stress is also at the root of many mental disorders including anxiety disorders. (Anxiety disorders will be discussed in Chapter 6.) Now, with the help of **Worksheet 2.2** (page 38), find out whether you experience any manifestations of chronic stress.

Worksheet 2.3 (page 39) has been designed to help you reflect on your thoughts in general. Thoughts and ensuing emotions are the most powerful sources of stress and are unfortunately the least emphasized and understood phenomena.

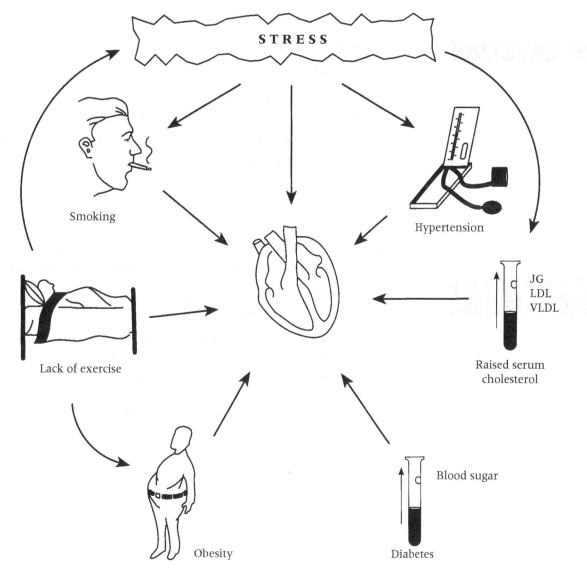

Figure 2.1 Relationship Between Stress and Heart Disease

stress and expectations

All of us will appreciate that the body has only a limited potential to process a few of the thoughts that come to our mind and that most of the unwanted, unprocessed thoughts contribute to our stress levels. Since we cannot do anything about the unwanted, unprocessed thoughts, we need to be selective and judiciously indulge in only those thoughts that we can process. The techniques to reduce these thoughts can only be acquired through proper conditioning of the mind over a period of time. This reduction in the number of unwanted thoughts will most certainly help in reducing our stress levels. How we interpret and label these thoughts is also important. Imagine a situation in which we observe our boss or teacher looking at us in an unusual way. It is easy for us to attribute this look as meaning that we are not doing well; thus this reaction is likely to be stressful and anxiety provoking. Interpretation of the same event as being due to the person being tired or having personal problems will not cause stress. Brooding over our thoughts or dwelling on our worries only adds to the tension in our

▓ Is it true that commitment is vital to the success of any task?

▓ Imagine all your past successes. Were you committed to the tasks?

▓ Does commitment reduce stress?

▓ If you are committed, would that fact reduce the chances of self-doubt, failure, and inefficiency? Would that improvement in turn reduce stress?

▓ What if you are not committed? Would that fact add to the confusion of roles that you perform? Would your confusion contribute to purposelessness and lack of direction?

True happiness, or *ananda* (Indian term), only arises if we focus on the present. If we can be happy now, then we have learned to be happy anytime. However, if we choose to believe that we will be happy:

▓ if ...   ▓ when ...   ▓ with ...   ▓ only if ...   ▓ in ...

then we are only making our happiness contingent on external things. We may become happy temporarily, but true happiness will elude us. True happiness, or *ananda,* is an internal feeling that cannot depend on any external object. This understanding has to be appreciated by us and also implemented in our daily life. We have to constantly keep reminding ourselves that *ananda* is an internal phenomenon not dependent on the outside world. We have to learn to be happy—"just happy"—and not happy "due to"...

body, which in turn creates the subjective feeling of uneasiness and leads to more anxious thoughts. Becoming excessively emotional about these thoughts is another factor that contributes to stress. Emotions or feelings are helpful, but if we become unduly emotional, then the emotions do not serve any purpose. Instead these emotions do more harm than good by stimulating the physiological processes and precipitating the stress response. This stress response drains away the vital energy needed by the body to perform important daily functions. Refer to Thoughts for Reflection 2.1, Commitment, and Thoughts for Reflection 2.2, True Happiness or Ananda, above.

Stress is also the result of our interactions with people, situations, and the environment. If we think about people and situations that contribute to our stress, we will find that people who are close to us and situations from which we expect to benefit are the things that contribute to most of our stress. This stress is tied into the inherent *expectations* that we have of these people and situations. Are these expectations realistic? Most of the time they are not.

We cannot become hermits or renounce the world and escape all stresses of life. However, we can learn to counteract our conventional response to stress by learning how to relax effectively and by reducing unwanted thoughts. These techniques help the body in attaining a state of balance, or *homeostasis*. Relaxation and thought modification restore our energy. Before we discuss the variety of stress management techniques, we have to enhance our awareness of the *type, frequency, intensity,* and *duration* of stress operating in our body. An awareness of any problem is certainly the first step toward a solution. Therefore, it is important for us to begin examining questions pertaining to *what, where, how,* and *when* before searching for a solution. Worksheets are aimed at enhancing your awareness of stress. Complete **Worksheets 2.4, 2.5,** and **2.6** (pages 40, 43, and 44, respectively).

sense of coherence

In 1970s Aaron Antonovsky (1979, 1987) presented the concept of sense of coherence. If a person has higher sense of coherence then he or she can cope better with stress. There are three components to this concept: (1) *comprehensibility* or the perception of stressors in a way such that they make cognitive sense and have structure, consistency, order, clarity and predictability; (2) *manageability* or the belief that one has the resources to control the demands posed by the stressors, and (3) *meaningfulness* or the belief that the stressors are worthy of commitment and engagement. **Worksheet 2.7** (page 50) helps us identify our level of sense of coherence. Take some time to complete it.

CHAPTER REVIEW

summary points

○ In addition to knowledge, for any change to occur, enhanced awareness is essential.

○ Components of the health belief model, which explains and predicts behavior change, are perceived susceptibility, perceived severity, perceived benefits, perceived barriers, cues to action, and self-efficacy.

○ Stress affects all of us. We all experience acute and chronic manifestations of stress.

○ Acute manifestations of stress are either predominantly in the body or primarily in the mind. For some, there may be a mixed reaction of both the body and mind.

○ Diseases such as hypertension, coronary heart disease, stroke, migraine headaches, peptic ulcers, arthritis, colitis, diarrhea, asthma, cardiac arrhythmias, sexual problems, circulatory problems, muscle tension, allergies, backache, temporomandibular joint syndrome, and cancer have been found to be associated with stress.

○ Maintaining a daily observation of stress in our lives is the first and foremost step in dealing with stress.

○ Commitment to alleviating stress is a vital prerequisite for initiating stress management programs.

important terms defined

ananda: A Sanskrit word denoting absolute joy, bliss, happiness, peace, or communion with totality.

cues to action: A component of the health belief model that implies precipitating forces that make a person feel the need to take action.

expectancies: A construct from the social cognitive theory that means the values that a person places on the anticipated outcome as a result of engaging in the chosen behavior.

expectations: A construct from the social cognitive theory that implies anticipations that a person has about the possible outcomes as a result of engaging in a desired behavior.

perceived barriers: A set of beliefs from the health belief model concerning actual and imagined costs in adhering to a preventive behavior.

perceived benefits: A set of beliefs from the health belief model that means how strongly a person believes about possible good things that will result if one engaged in a preventive behavior.

perceived severity: A component of the health belief model that implies the extent of harm a person may have to endure due to a disease or harmful state as a result of engaging in a particular behavior.

perceived susceptibility: A set of beliefs from the health belief model that means how strongly a person believes regarding the acquisition of a disease or a harmful state as a result of engaging in a particular behavior.

self-control: A construct from the social cognitive theory that implies explicit and specific goal setting for behavior change.

self-efficacy: A construct from social cognitive theory and the health belief model that describes a behavior and situation-specific confidence a person has in his or her ability to perform a behavior.

situational perception: A construct from the social cognitive theory that entails how an individual looks at the environment and interprets it.

websites to explore

FUTURE HEALTH

www.futurehealth.org

This is the website of an organization founded in 1978 as a resource center for information about instruments, books, supplies, training programs, conferences, and websites related to stress.

■ Using the website, explore the recent conferences and other events related to stress. Which one would you like to participate in, and why? Can you also get more web-based information on the chosen event and have virtual participation if not real?

KANSAS STATE UNIVERSITY COUNSELING SERVICES

www.ksu.edu/counseling

This website is put up by Kansas State University Counseling Services.

▤ Visit this website and read the information. Do you have a counseling center at your university? Plan to find out more information about the services offered by your university's center through a personal visit. Summarize the services offered by the center in the form of a brochure.

MENTAL HEALTH AMERICA

www.nmha.org

This is the website of Mental Health America (MHA). Established in 1909 by former psychiatric patient Clifford W. Beers, MHA is among the oldest nonprofit organizations. Today, it has more than 340 affiliates and strives to improve the mental health of all Americans, particularly the 54 million individuals with mental disorders, through advocacy, education, research, and service.

▤ This website provides tips for college students. Which aspect of these tips do you agree with, and why? Which aspects of these tips do you not agree with, and why?

SEARCH ENGINE

www.google.com

There are millions of documents on the web. Search engines allow you to enter key words and identify all the documents that match those key words. There are a plethora of such engines. For further details on search engines, check out http://www.searchenginewatch.com.

▤ Using the search engine Google, conduct a search on social cognitive theory and Albert Bandura. Using the information located from one or more websites, write a brief paper on the life and contributions of Bandura.

How Your Body Reacts to Acute Stress

Imagine yourself in a stressful situation. When you are feeling anxious or stressed, what do you typically experience? Check all the items that apply.

_____ 1. My heart starts to beat faster and pound harder.

_____ 2. I cannot prevent disturbing thoughts from entering my mind.

_____ 3. My hands become cold and clammy.

_____ 4. I keep brooding on trivial thoughts over and over again.

_____ 5. I begin to sweat profusely.

_____ 6. I lose the power to concentrate and function effectively.

_____ 7. I develop irritable bowel syndrome or diarrhea.

_____ 8. I cannot make decisions and feel horrible.

_____ 9. I cannot sit still and nervously pace up and down.

_____ 10. I imagine the worst possible scenario and cannot stop thinking about it.

_____ 11. My abdomen begins to hurt.

_____ 12. I feel the world around me is crashing and I have lost all control.

_____ 13. I feel restless.

_____ 14. I imagine horrifying scenes that keep me disturbed for a long time.

_____ 15. My body gets stiff, and I am immobilized.

_____ 16. I think of leaving everything and just running away.

_____ 17. I have a feeling of "butterflies" in my stomach.

_____ 18. I want the situation to end favorably as soon as possible but am not sure.

_____ 19. I feel tired and exhausted after some time.

_____ 20. I develop a headache.

FEEDBACK ON WORKSHEET 2.1

Count the even-numbered and odd-numbered responses separately.

- Odd-numbered responses = _____
- Even-numbered responses = _____

If you have scored more even-numbered responses than odd, then you tend to respond to stress with your *mind*. This result also signifies that you are likely to derive greater relaxation by indulging in the activities of mind like meditation, any interesting hobby, and so on. If you have scored more odd-numbered responses, then your *body* tends to respond more to stress. People who respond to stress by having symptoms in the body generally require systematic physical activity like aerobic exercise, progressive muscle relaxation, and other such techniques. If you have a near equal mixture of even- and odd-numbered responses, then you respond to stress in a *mixed* fashion. A combination of mind relaxation and physical activities is likely to benefit you in relieving stress.

_____

Note: Based upon personal discussions with Peter R. Kovacek, Henry Ford Hospital, Detroit, MI, 1981.

Do You Suffer From Chronic Stress?

Check all the items that apply to you.

_____ 1. I frequently suffer from a burning sensation in the upper abdominal region.

_____ 2. I often belch and have difficulty digesting food.

_____ 3. I often have backaches or joint pains.

_____ 4. I frequently suffer from headaches.

_____ 5. I sometimes have chest pain.

_____ 6. I have been diagnosed as having heart disease or hypertension.

_____ 7. I have had a stroke.

_____ 8. I frequently develop cold hands and feet.

_____ 9. I frequently have diarrhea and loose bowel movements, especially when I am anxious.

_____ 10. I suffer from a great deal of anxiety.

_____

Note: Consider seeking medical attention if symptoms identified above persist.

FEEDBACK ON WORKSHEET 2.2

If you have checked any of the items, you are likely to be suffering from the effects of chronic stress. Don't worry! It is still not too late to change your lifestyle.

If you have checked items 1 and 2, then you are a likely candidate for a *peptic ulcer*, which is precipitated and aggravated by stress. Item 3 pertains to *backache* and *arthritis*, which have been associated with chronic stress. Item 4 refers to *migraine* and *tension headaches*, which are also a result of stress. Items 5–7 pertain to *coronary heart disease* and *hypertension*. Item 8 refers to *circulatory*

problems, which are stress related. Item 9 indicates *diarrhea* and *colitis*, which have been related to stress. Finally, item 10 pertains to generalized anxiety disorder, which is also a result of chronic stress.

If you are young, it is likely that you may not have checked any of the items. This result only indicates that you have not yet been affected by the harmful effects of stress. Therefore, it is all the more reason for you to practice stress reduction, prevention, and management techniques.

Thought Identification

For the next 15 minutes, leave aside everything you have been doing and try to write down *all* the thoughts that come into your mind starting in the space provided and then on additional sheets of paper. Be sure to write down everything, even if it may appear trivial or unimportant.

_____

_____

_____

_____

_____

_____

_____

_____

_____

_____

_____

_____

_____

_____

FEEDBACK ON WORKSHEET 2.3

Notice how many thoughts have come to your mind in such a short period of time—just 15 minutes. Count these thoughts. Multiply this figure by 4 to determine the number of thoughts that come to your mind in an hour. Calculate the total number of thoughts that come to your mind in a year and in 75 years.

Number of thoughts in 15 minutes: $(A) = $ _____
Number of thoughts in 1 hour: $(B) = (A \times 4) = $ _____
Number of thoughts in 1 day: $(C) = (B \times 24) = $ _____
Number of thoughts in 1 year: $(D) = (C \times 365) = $ _____
Number of thoughts in 75 years: $(E) = (D \times 75) = $ _____

This is a simplistic calculation. For the sake of simplicity we have included all the time in the day. However, when we are deeply engrossed in certain tasks or when we are in a deep sleep, the number of thoughts decreases. It needs to be noted that in light sleep, while dreaming, the frequency of thoughts increases. In essence, this pattern may have a canceling-out effect. Therefore, these calculations may be close to accurate.

Thus, you can appreciate that in your lifetime you generate a large number of thoughts and that only a few of these are relevant and need to be processed. This realization will help you to reduce your stress and lead a productive life.

Stress Awareness Log

PRINCIPLES

A daily record of stressors can serve as a valuable tool in learning to cope with stress. Keeping a stress log is an excellent tool for this purpose. The stress awareness log serves three important purposes:

1. It helps familiarize you with how you *react* to stress.

2. It helps you rule out any symptoms that are not related to stress.

3. It helps you establish some baseline data and develop your goals for reducing stress.

Initially, maintaining this stress awareness log may appear complicated and time-consuming. Once you have used these log sheets for a few days and have become familiar with this means of record keeping, it will take only a few minutes of your time every day.

The information that you record on the stress log is for your use only. You need not share it with anyone. It is important that you be *candid and honest* with yourself in filling out these log sheets. If your daily experiences remain unclear, then the means for finding appropriate solutions will also be hazy. It is important that you maintain the log sheets for *at least five consecutive days*. Try to include a weekend in your recordings, as we normally tend to behave differently over weekends and sometimes this difference may contribute to your stress.

The most important part of the stress awareness log is for you to maintain it *conscientiously*. It is a very effective tool to help you identify ways in which you react to stress. However, unless you maintain it accurately and work at it, it will be of no value and may even contribute to increasing your stress levels. The more information you put into this stress awareness log, the more you will benefit in the long run.

RECORDING INSTRUCTIONS

Under the headings listed in the following paragraphs, you should make a record on the log sheets as described.

■ *Time of day* includes a serial record of time for each event chronologically. You need to use one log sheet per day. Photocopy the sheet provided in order to record your information for a minimum of five days.

■ *Signals* are indicators, manifestations, signs, symptoms, responses, and reactions (e.g., *physical*—headache, muscle tension, perspiration, palpitation, or rapid heart rate; *mental*—loss of attention span, poor concentration, effect on memory, or impaired judgment; *behavioral*—inability to interact with others, uncontrolled anger, or reduced job performance).

■ *Stressors* are events that can be looked upon as "inputs" originating from your thoughts, feelings, situations, and the environment. If the event causes stress or interferes with your ability to accomplish daily tasks, then it is a stressor. It is also important to consider different intensity levels of various stressors.

■ *How am I dealing with the stressors?* In this section you can record techniques and mechanisms, if any, that you have been using in handling the stressors. It would also be worthwhile to record the time of day the technique was used and whether or not it made a difference.

■ *How effective have I been? What else can I do?* This section includes whether or not you were able to work with the stressor in a satisfactory way and if the means of resolution worked. Other comments, if necessary, may be added in this section.

Record on the sheets for at least four to five consecutive days. You may also prepare a brief summary statement of the information entered on your log sheets, if you need to share it with someone else or if you want concise information for greater insight.

Stress Awareness Log *(cont'd)*

Day 1 Day and Date: _____

Time of Day	Signals	Stressor	How Am I Dealing With the Stressors?	How Effective Have I Been? What Else Can I Do?

Day 2 Day and Date: _____

Time of Day	Signals	Stressor	How Am I Dealing With the Stressors?	How Effective Have I Been? What Else Can I Do?

Day 3 Day and Date: _____

Time of Day	Signals	Stressor	How Am I Dealing With the Stressors?	How Effective Have I Been? What Else Can I Do?

Day 4 Day and Date: _____

Time of Day	Signals	Stressor	How Am I Dealing With the Stressors?	How Effective Have I Been? What Else Can I Do?

Day 5 Day and Date: _____

Time of Day	Signals	Stressor	How Am I Dealing With the Stressors?	How Effective Have I Been? What Else Can I Do?

FEEDBACK ON WORKSHEET 2.4

A stress awareness log is an excellent tool that provides you with accurate feedback about your present stress levels. If it is maintained carefully and honestly, it generates useful insight into your behavior and provides an important basis for initiating change in your lifestyle. It also helps you see unhealthy lifestyles that jeopardize your health. It is an important first step to initiate any subsequent changes.

To interpret the information from the Stress Awareness Log, be objective. Critically appraise your behavior and identify the changes that can be easily and effectively incorporated into your daily lifestyle. In subsequent chapters of this workbook, these changes are discussed step by step.

Stress and Tension Test

Reflect on the past month and try to answer the following questions as honestly as possible. Circle your responses.

		Always	Often	Sometimes	Rarely
1.	I feel tense, anxious, and uptight.	3	2	1	0
2.	I cannot stop worrying at night and during my leisure time.	3	2	1	0
3.	I have headaches, backache, and pain in the shoulder or neck.	3	2	1	0
4.	My sleep is disrupted, and I usually keep getting up while sleeping.	3	2	1	0
5.	People around me tend to cause stress for me and make me irritable.	3	2	1	0
6.	I tend to eat, drink, and/or smoke in response to my stress and anxiety.	3	2	1	0
7.	I do not feel refreshed in the mornings and am normally tired, lethargic, and exhausted during the day.	3	2	1	0
8.	I find it difficult to concentrate on the tasks and activities that I am supposed to perform.	3	2	1	0
9.	I have to use tranquilizers, sedatives, or other drugs to relax.	3	2	1	0
10.	I cannot find time to relax.	3	2	1	0
11.	I have too many deadlines to meet, and I fall behind in accomplishing them.	3	2	1	0

Note: From John W. Farquhar, *The American way of life need not be hazardous to your health,* revised edition. Reprinted with permission from John W. Farquhar..

FEEDBACK ON WORKSHEET 2.5

If you have a score over 22, you certainly have been experiencing high stress levels and you need to relax. You may also require help from others. If your score is below 22, then you may not be stressed as much at present, but in order to continue being relaxed and stress free, you need to practice techniques of stress management, reduction, and prevention.

Personal Stress Test

This test is designed to help you assess the impact of stress at this point in your life. Your response to each statement can provide information to help you deal with stress. This test does not assess physical, mental, or emotional illness. It is designed for normal, healthy individuals who want to control stress in a positive manner and enjoy life more.

Fill out the test when you are certain not to be interrupted. Respond to each statement using the scale at the left side of the page. There are no right or wrong answers. Some statements may seem hard to respond to because they are subjective. If none of the available responses appears to fit perfectly, pick the one closest to the way you feel. Do not consult the test feedback sheet until you have finished the test. While it is not mandatory to respond to any item you find objectionable, results from completed tests are more accurate. Thus, you should complete the entire test.

Circle the letter to the right of each statement that best describes you and how often you feel that way. Answer each statement honestly.

PROFILE CODE:

- N = almost never
- R = rarely
- S = sometimes
- O = often
- A = almost always

PROFILE QUESTIONS

1.	There are situations in which I cannot be myself.	N	R	S	O	A
2.	I have the stamina and endurance I need.	N	R	S	O	A
3.	I worry about how things will turn out.	N	R	S	O	A
4.	I am happy and content.	N	R	S	O	A
5.	I feel motivated to do things.	N	R	S	O	A
6.	I feel sad and down in the dumps.	N	R	S	O	A
7.	I feel in control of my appetite.	N	R	S	O	A
8.	I am sluggish and lack energy.	N	R	S	O	A
9.	I feel loved by someone important to me.	N	R	S	O	A
10.	I feel I am well organized and clearheaded.	N	R	S	O	A
11.	My life lacks stimulation.	N	R	S	O	A
12.	Day-to-day living is monotonous for me.	N	R	S	O	A
13.	I accomplish things that are important to me.	N	R	S	O	A
14.	I feel physically strong and capable.	N	R	S	O	A
15.	I fit in well with the people around me.	N	R	S	O	A
16.	I feel resentment about things that have happened to me in the past.	N	R	S	O	A
17.	I enjoy being with the people around me.	N	R	S	O	A
18.	There is a difference between how I think I should be and how I am.	N	R	S	O	A

Personal Stress Test (cont'd)

		N	R	S	O	A
19.	My stomach bothers me.	N	R	S	O	A
20.	I am lonely.	N	R	S	O	A
21.	I think I am living life to the fullest.	N	R	S	O	A
22.	I have the standard of living I deserve.	N	R	S	O	A
23.	I feel excluded by people.	N	R	S	O	A
24.	I have difficulty concentrating.	N	R	S	O	A
25.	I feel relaxed.	N	R	S	O	A
26.	I feel guilty about eating.	N	R	S	O	A
27.	I have a clear conscience.	N	R	S	O	A
28.	I have aches and pains.	N	R	S	O	A
29.	I would like to start all over.	N	R	S	O	A
30.	I have pleasant feelings.	N	R	S	O	A
31.	It is hard for me to get close to people.	N	R	S	O	A
32.	I worry about my weight.	N	R	S	O	A
33.	I feel I belong.	N	R	S	O	A
34.	I feel like I am part of a family.	N	R	S	O	A
35.	My life is dull and uninteresting.	N	R	S	O	A
36.	Things that happen to me are unfair.	N	R	S	O	A
37.	I can remember important things.	N	R	S	O	A
38.	I feel nervous or upset.	N	R	S	O	A
39.	I feel good about my eating habits.	N	R	S	O	A
40.	I get what I want.	N	R	S	O	A

FEEDBACK ON WORKSHEET 2.6

1. Place your Personal Stress Test alongside the following answer key.

2. This answer key is divided into ten categories.

3. To find the score for each item, carefully circle the number below the letter you chose on your stress test.

4. Enter the score for each question in the proper bracket in the Total Points column.

5. Then total the score for each category on the following page.

Note: The order of the items on this answer key is not the same as the order on the test.

(continued)

Stress Factor	Question Number	Scoring Key					Total Points
		N	R	S	O	A	
1. Physical condition	2	5	4	3	2	1	_____
	8	1	2	3	4	5	_____
	14	5	4	3	2	1	_____
	28	1	2	3	4	5	_____
						Subtotal	_____
2. Mental performance	3	1	2	3	4	5	_____
	10	5	4	3	2	1	_____
	24	1	2	3	4	5	_____
	37	5	4	3	2	1	_____
						Subtotal	_____
3. Emotional relaxation	19	1	2	3	4	5	_____
	25	5	4	3	2	1	_____
	30	5	4	3	2	1	_____
	38	1	2	3	4	5	_____
						Subtotal	_____
4. Weight control and image	7	5	4	3	2	1	_____
	26	1	2	3	4	5	_____
	32	1	2	3	4	5	_____
	39	5	4	3	2	1	_____
						Subtotal	_____
5. Sense of belonging	15	5	4	3	2	1	_____
	20	1	2	3	4	5	_____
	33	5	4	3	2	1	_____
	34	5	4	3	2	1	_____
						Subtotal	_____

Stress Factor	Question Number	Scoring Key					Total Points
		N	R	S	O	A	
6. Sense of relationship	9	5	4	3	2	1	_____
	17	5	4	3	2	1	_____
	23	1	2	3	4	5	_____
	31	1	2	3	4	5	_____
						Subtotal	_____
7. Sense of satisfaction	4	5	4	3	2	1	_____
	21	5	4	3	2	1	_____
	29	1	2	3	4	5	_____
	35	1	2	3	4	5	_____
						Subtotal	_____
8. Sense of integrity	1	1	2	3	4	5	_____
	13	5	4	3	2	1	_____
	18	1	2	3	4	5	_____
	27	5	4	3	2	1	_____
						Subtotal	_____
9. Sense of justice	16	1	2	3	4	5	_____
	22	5	4	3	2	1	_____
	36	1	2	3	4	5	_____
	40	5	4	3	2	1	_____
						Subtotal	_____
10. Sense of stimulation	5	5	4	3	2	1	_____
	6	1	2	3	4	5	_____
	11	1	2	3	4	5	_____
	12	1	2	3	4	5	_____
						Subtotal	_____

Now transfer these scores where indicated on the following sheet to obtain your Personal Stress Profile.

(continued)

Transfer the subtotal scores calculated on the preceding pages for each category under the subtotal scores column below. Then, place an X on the adjoining scale. This scale visually reveals your areas of low, moderate, and high stress in these categories.

PERSONAL STRESS PROFILE

		SCALE					
		Low		Moderate		High	
Stress Profile Factor	Subtotal Scores	0	7	8	15	16	20
1. Physical condition	_____						
2. Mental performance	_____						
3. Emotional relaxation	_____						
4. Weight control and image	_____						
5. Sense of belonging	_____						
6. Sense of relationship	_____						
7. Sense of satisfaction	_____						
8. Sense of integrity	_____						
9. Sense of justice	_____						
10. Sense of stimulation	_____						

INTERPRETATION OF SCORES

	Factor	COMMON INDICATORS		
		High 16–20 (poor coping)	Moderate 8–15 (dissatisfaction)	Low 0–7 (good coping)
1.	Physical condition	▪ Aches, pains ▪ Fatigue ▪ Listlessness ▪ Illness prone	▪ Energy level fluctuations ▪ Little stamina	▪ Stamina ▪ Strength ▪ Active
2.	Mental performance	▪ Forgets details ▪ Worries a lot ▪ Ruminates	▪ Confusion ▪ Mind vacillates ▪ Details escape	▪ Clarity ▪ Solves problems ▪ Concentrate
3.	Emotional relaxation	▪ Tense ▪ Nervous ▪ Anxious ▪ Sleeplessness ▪ Stomach churnings	▪ Irritable ▪ Inner turmoil ▪ Some tension	▪ Calm ▪ Confident ▪ Relaxed

Factor	COMMON INDICATORS		
	High 16–20 (poor coping)	Moderate 8–15 (dissatisfaction)	Low 0–7 (good coping)
4. Weight control and image	▪ Eats more ▪ Disappointed with image	▪ Eats too much or too little ▪ Not satisfied with image	▪ Eats when hungry ▪ Balanced diet
5. Sense of belonging	▪ Alienated ▪ Loneliness ▪ Separation	▪ Close to only a few ▪ Distant with others	▪ Common bonds with many ▪ Comfortable with others
6. Sense of relationship	▪ Tense relations ▪ Withdrawal	▪ Shares little about self ▪ Few inquiries about others ▪ Unpredictable	▪ Strong friendships ▪ Long-term relations
7. Sense of satisfaction	▪ Wanting to start life over	▪ Unsure ▪ Questions ▪ Disinterested ▪ Discontent	▪ Happy ▪ Contented ▪ Enthusiasm ▪ Fulfillment
8. Sense of integrity	▪ Reserved ▪ Unsure ▪ Expedient	▪ Inconsistent ▪ Regrets behavior ▪ Attitude of martyrdom	▪ Acts on priorities ▪ Pride in accomplishment
9. Sense of justice	▪ Resentment ▪ Anger ▪ Incapable	▪ Roll with punches ▪ Questions	▪ Control ▪ Fairness ▪ Balance
10. Sense of stimulation	▪ Monotony ▪ Boredom ▪ Laziness	▪ Moderate interest in life ▪ Future has appeal	▪ Enthusiasm ▪ Motivation ▪ Takes initiative

Note: From *Coping with stress* by Medicine Shoppe International, Inc., 1985, St. Louis, MO: Medicine Shoppe International, Inc. Copyright 1985 Medicine Shoppe International, Inc. Used with permission.

WORKSHEET 2.7

This worksheet is available online at www.pearsonhighered.com/romas.

Sense of Coherence Test

Sense of coherence has three components: Comprehensibility (C), Manageability (MA), and Meaningfulness (ME). In the questionnaire the items that tap into each of these components are marked by the initials on the left side of each item.

The questionnaire also has four facets: A. Modality (with 3 elements: 1. instrumental; 2. cognitive; 3. affective); B. Source (with 3 elements: 1. internal; 2. external; 3. both); C. Demand (with 3 elements: 1 concrete; 2. diffuse; 3 abstract); D. Time (with 3 elements: 1. past; 2. present; 3. future). These elements are also indicated by four numbers on the left side of each item. Also R is marked on 13 items, which signifies that before calculating the score these items should be reversed and 13 items have been marked with an asterisk (*). These asterisk-marked items constitute the short version SOC-13.

1. C R 1312 When you talk to people, do you have the feeling that they don't understand you?

| 1 | 2 | 3 | 4 | 5 | 6 | 7 |

never have this feeling   always have this feeling

2. MA 1111 In the past, when you had to do something which depended upon cooperation with others, did you have the feeling that it:

| 1 | 2 | 3 | 4 | 5 | 6 | 7 |

surely wouldn't get done   surely would get done

3. C 1322 Think of the people with whom you come into contact daily, aside from the ones to whom you feel closest. How well do you know most of them?

| 1 | 2 | 3 | 4 | 5 | 6 | 7 |

you feel that they're strangers   you know them very well

*4. ME R 1222 Do you have the feeling that you don't really care about what goes on around you?

| 1 | 2 | 3 | 4 | 5 | 6 | 7 |

very seldom or never   very often

*5. C R 1221 Has it happened in the past that you were surprised by the behavior of people whom you thought you knew well?

| 1 | 2 | 3 | 4 | 5 | 6 | 7 |

never happened   always happened

*6. MA R 1221 Has it happened that people whom you counted on disappointed you?

| 1 | 2 | 3 | 4 | 5 | 6 | 7 |

never happened   always happened

7. ME R 2332 Life is:

| 1 | 2 | 3 | 4 | 5 | 6 | 7 |

full of interest   completely routine

Sense of Coherence Test *(cont'd)*

*8. ME 2331 Until now your life has had:

1	2	3	4	5	6	7

no clear goals or purpose at all   very clear goals and purpose

*9. MA 1221 Do you have the feeling that you're being treated unfairly?

1	2	3	4	5	6	7

very often   very seldom or never

10. C 2331 In the past ten years your life has been:

1	2	3	4	5	6	7

full changes without your knowing   completely consistent and clear
what will happen next

11. ME R 1313 Most of the things you do in future will probably be:

1	2	3	4	5	6	7

completely fascinating   deadly boring

*12. C 2232 Do you have the feeling that you are in an unfamiliar situation and don't know what to do?

1	2	3	4	5	6	7

very often   very seldom or never

13. MA R 2332 What best describes how you see life?

1	2	3	4	5	6	7

one can always find a   there is no solution to painful things in life
solution in life

14. ME R 2132 When you think about your life, you very often:

1	2	3	4	5	6	7

feel how good it is to be alive   ask yourself why you exist at all

15. C 1112 When you face a difficult problem, the choice of a solution is:

1	2	3	4	5	6	7

always confusing and hard   always completely clear
to find

*16. ME R 1312 Doing the things you do every day is:

1	2	3	4	5	6	7

a source of deep pleasure and satisfaction   a source of pain and boredom

(continued)

Sense of Coherence Test (cont'd)

17. C   2333 Your life in the future will probably be:

| 1 | 2 | 3 | 4 | 5 | 6 | 7 |

full of changes without your knowing   completely consistent and clear
what will happen next

18. MA   3211 When something unpleasant happened in the past your tendency was:

| 1 | 2 | 3 | 4 | 5 | 6 | 7 |

"to eat yourself up" about it   to say "ok , that's that, I have to
live with it and go on

19. C   2122 Do you have very mixed-up feelings and ideas?

| 1 | 2 | 3 | 4 | 5 | 6 | 7 |

very often   very seldom or never

20. MA R 1113 When you do something that gives you a good feeling:

| 1 | 2 | 3 | 4 | 5 | 6 | 7 |

It's certain that you'll go on feeling good   it's certain that something will happen to spoil the feeling

21. C   3122 Does it happen that you have feelings inside you would rather not feel?

| 1 | 2 | 3 | 4 | 5 | 6 | 7 |

very often   very seldom or never

22. ME 2333 You anticipate that your personal life in the future will be:

| 1 | 2 | 3 | 4 | 5 | 6 | 7 |

totally without meaning or purpose   full of meaning and purpose

23. MA R 1223 Do you think that there will *always* be people whom you'll be able to count on in the future?

| 1 | 2 | 3 | 4 | 5 | 6 | 7 |

you're certain there will be   you doubt there will be

24. C   2233 Does it happen that you have the feeling that you don't know exactly what's about to happen?

| 1 | 2 | 3 | 4 | 5 | 6 | 7 |

very often   very seldom or never

*25. MA R 3131 Many people — even those a strong character – sometimes feel like sad sacks (losers) in certain situations. How often have you felt this way in the past?

| 1 | 2 | 3 | 4 | 5 | 6 | 7 |

never   very often

Sense of Coherence Test (cont'd)

*26. C 1211 When something happened, have you generally found that:

1	2	3	4	5	6	7

you overestimated or
underestimated

you saw things in the right its   proportion
importance

27. MA R 1313 When you think of difficulties you are likely to face in important aspects of your life, do you have the feeling that:

1	2	3	4	5	6	7

you will always succeed
in overcoming

you won't succeed in overcoming   the difficulties
the difficulties

*28. ME 1212 How often do you have the feeling that there is little meaning in the things you do in your daily life?

1	2	3	4	5	6	7

very often   very seldom or never

*29. MA 3122 How often do you have feelings that you're not sure you can keep under control?

1	2	3	4	5	6	7

very often   very seldom or never

FEEDBACK ON WORKSHEET 2.7

Reverse the scores on 13 items with the R. Then total all the points. If your score is over 100 points then that indicates higher sense of coherence. The higher the score, the stronger is the sense of coherence. You can also check your scores in each of the three areas constituting sense of coherence. If you have less time you can do only the items marked with the asterisk and your score of 45 or higher will denote higher sense of coherence.

Source. Antonovsky, A. (1987). *Unraveling the mystery of health. How people manage stress and stay well* (pp. 189–194). San Francisco: Jossey-Bass Publishers.

references and further readings

Antonovsky, A. (1979). *Health, stress, and coping.* San Francisco: Jossey-Bass.

Antonovsky, A. (1987). *Unraveling the mystery of health: How people manage stress and stay well.* San Francisco: Jossey-Bass.

Bandura, A. (Ed.). (1995). *Self-efficacy in changing societies.* New York: Cambridge University Press.

Bandura, A. (2004). Health promotion by social cognitive means. *Health Education & Behavior, 31,* 143–164.

Becker, M. H. (1974). The health belief model and personal health behavior. *Health Education Monographs, 2,* 324–473.

Farquhar, J. W. (1979). *The American way of life need not be hazardous to your health.* New York: Norton.

Girdano, D. A., Everly, G. S., Jr., & Dusek, D. E. (2012). *Controlling stress and tension: A holistic approach* (9th ed.). Englewood Cliffs, NJ: Prentice Hall.

Glanz, K., Rimer, B. K., & Viswanath, K. (2002). *Health behavior and health education: Theory, research, and practice* (4th ed.). San Francisco: Jossey-Bass.

Green, L. W., & Kreuter, M. W. (2005). *Health promotion planning: An educational and environmental approach* (4th ed.). Boston: McGraw-Hill.

Greenberg, J. S. (2010). *Comprehensive stress management* (12th ed.). Boston: McGraw-Hill.

Hamet, P., & Tremblay, J. (2002). Genetic determinants of the stress response in cardiovascular disease. *Metabolism, 51,* 15–24.

Hochbaum, G. M. (1958). *Public participation in medical screening programs: A sociopsychological study.* PHS Publication No. 572. Washington, DC: Government Printing Office.

Kubzansky, L. D., & Koenen, K. C. (2009). Is posttraumatic stress disorder related to development of heart disease? An update. *Cleveland Clinic Journal of Medicine, 76* (Suppl 2), S60-S65.

Labarthe, D. R., & Roccella, E. J. (1993). High blood pressure. In R. C. Brownson, P. L. Remington, & J. R. Davis (Eds.), *Chronic disease epidemiology and control* (p. 109). Washington, DC: American Public Health Association.

Matthews, K. A., & Gump, B. B. (2002). Chronic work stress and marital dissolution increase risk of post trial mortality in men from the Multiple Risk Factor Intervention Trial. *Archives of Internal Medicine, 162,* 309–315.

Rice, P. L. (1999). *Stress and health* (3rd ed.). Pacific Grove, CA: Wadsworth.

Sharma, M., & Romas, J. A. (2012). *Theoretical foundations of health education and health promotion* (2nd ed.). Sudbury, MA: Jones and Bartlett.

Smith, J. C. (1993). *Understanding stress and coping.* New York: Macmillan.

Von Kanel, R., Mills, P. J., Fainman, C., & Dimsdale, J. E. (2001). Effects of psychological stress and psychiatric disorders on blood coagulation and fibrimolysis: A biobehavioral pathway to coronary artery disease? *Psychosomatic Medicine, 63,* 531–544.

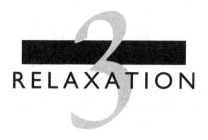

RELAXATION

" Make relaxation a part of your life. "

what is relaxation?

The word *relax* is derived from the Latin word *relaxare*, meaning "to loosen." Indeed, relaxation implies loosening up or letting go. By this process of relaxing or loosening, all living beings consolidate and restore energy that has been lost in daily activities. Therefore, relaxation is vital for the normal functioning of any living organism. Relaxation techniques form the core of all stress management programs. When our bodies are functioning normally, we derive relaxation through sleep.

sleep

We all sleep. Without sleep we cannot live, although there may be some exceptions. Sleep accomplishes two vital functions—*conservation of energy* and *restoration of energy* (Shapiro & Flanigan, 1993). Sleep deprivation causes impairments in cognitive functions (McCoy & Strecker, 2011; Zhang & Liu, 2008). Sleep follows a circadian rhythm, or a daily pattern (Mong et al., 2011; Krauchi & Wirz-Justice, 2001; Schulz, 2007). Expenditure of energy is mainly measured by the metabolic rate (in simple terms, the rate of conversion of ingested food into energy useful for the body), which is raised during the day and reduced during the night (particularly during sleep) by 5 to 25 percent (Shapiro & Flanigan, 1993).

Physiologically, sleep is composed of two phases (Fuller, Gooley, & Saper, 2006; LeBow et al., 2002):

1. *Non-REM (non-rapid eye movement) sleep*

The non-REM sleep phase is characterized by four stages:

- *Stage 1* is a light, drowsy phase of non-REM sleep (the transition from wakefulness to sleep). This stage generally lasts one to seven minutes (Fuller et al., 2006) and is associated with a low arousal threshold (Markov & Goldman, 2006). Electroencephalography is a scientific method that helps gauge the electrical impulses within the brain with the help of electrodes placed over the scalp. Normally, if this electroencephalogram (EEG) recording is done during the awake state, when our mind and senses are working, then this recording will manifest *beta waves* (fast waves at a rhythm of 14–40 cycles per second). As drowsiness sets in, the frequency of beta waves starts to recede.

- *Stage 2* is the first real stage of sleep, which is characterized by *spindles* and *K complexes* on an EEG. This stage lasts for about 10 to 25 minutes in the first sleep cycle and gradually increases in length with each subsequent cycle. It comprises between 45 percent and 55 percent of total non-REM sleep (Hirshkowitz, 2004). During this stage of non-REM sleep, the EEG will record *alpha waves* (slower waves at 8–13 cycles per second). In this stage the mind comes to a peaceful state.

- *Stages 3 and 4* are known as "slow-wave sleep." In these stages of non-REM-phase sleep, the mind becomes subtler, and the EEG records *theta waves* (4–7 cycles per second). In extremely deep sleep or coma, the EEG records *delta waves* (near 1 cycle per second).

2. *REM (rapid eye movement) sleep*

REM sleep is the phase during which most dreaming happens. It occurs approximately 90 minutes after the person falls asleep. During this stage the mind functions at alpha and beta waves. From a stress perspective, during this phase a person does not actually become relaxed. However, this is still an important phase of sleep.

There is a cycle of non-REM and REM sleep throughout the night. As night progresses, the episodes of non-REM sleep become shorter, and those of the REM phase of sleep longer. Most slow-wave sleep occurs during the first third of the night, and most REM sleep occurs during the last third (Kalat, 1988).

How much sleep do we need? It depends on age. Infants require about 16–18 hours of sleep per day. Children need 12–16 hours of sleep. Adolescents require 9–10 hours of sleep. Adults need 7–8 hours of sleep. In older adults, sleep is decreased. Epidemiological studies have shown that both less (<7 hours) and more (>8 hours) sleep is associated with increased rates of morbidity (Cumberbatch et al., 2011; Hall et al., 2008) and mortality (Hublin, Partinen, Koskenvuo, & Kaprio, 2007).

However, when we are stressed, our normal biorhythm is altered, and our sleep pattern is disturbed. Therefore, our bodies cannot conserve and restore the lost energy. This altered biorhythm in turn adds to the stress, and a vicious cycle is set. If this disturbed sleep pattern is not changed or relaxation methods are not used, complete balance and harmony are disrupted. College students are particularly vulnerable to disturbances related to sleep.

It may even be the other way around. If we sleep less, for reasons of over-work or not being able to find enough time, our biorhythm becomes altered. Therefore, the body needs other forms of relaxation in order to conserve and restore lost energy.

If sleep is disturbed over a relatively long period of time, it can lead to sleep disorders. There are several kinds of sleep disorders. A population-based study by Bixler and colleagues (1979) found the overall prevalence of current or previous sleep disorders in adults to be as high as 52.1 percent. The 2005-2008 National Health and Nutrition Examination Survey (NHANES) by Centers for Disease Control and Prevention (CDC, 2011) found that 37.1 percent of adults slept for less than 7 hours. The most common sleep disorder is insomnia (Costa e Silva, 2006). Population-based estimates of the prevalence of insomnia in adults have varied considerably, from 10.2 percent (Ford & Kamerow, 1989) to 37.8 percent (Radecki & Brunton, 1993). According to DSM-IV, insomnia is associated with complaints about the quantity, quality, or timing of sleep more than three times a week for at least one month. Some other sleep disorders are:

○ *hypersomnia* (excessive sleepiness associated with difficulty in waking)

○ *narcolepsy* (excessive sleepiness that is typically associated with cataplexy—a sudden loss of muscle tone and paralysis of voluntary muscles that is associated with a strong emotion)

○ *sleep apnea* (repetitive episodes of upper airway obstruction during sleep)

○ *restless leg syndrome* (disagreeable leg sensations, usually prior to sleep onset, that cause an almost irresistible urge to move the legs)

○ *circadian rhythm disorders* (due to timing of sleep within the 24-hour day as a result of work shifts, jet lag, etc.)

○ *sleep talking* (uttering of speech or sounds during sleep without awareness of the event).

Sleep hygiene is an effective method to improve the quality and duration of sleep. Sleep hygiene is based on the assumption that behavioral and environmental factors can be altered to enhance sleep quality and duration (Stepanski & Wyatt, 2003). The following are some sleep hygiene practices:

1. Having a consistent time for sleeping and waking.

2. Avoiding long (1–2 hours) daytime naps.

3. Avoiding caffeine.

4. Avoiding alcohol.

5. Avoiding tobacco.

6. Avoiding large meals close to bed time.

7. Exercising 4–6 hours before sleeping but not right before sleeping (no exercise 2–4 hours before sleeping).

8. Using passive heating such as hot bath hours before sleep.

9. Eliminating light and noise sources from the bedroom.

10. Controlling temperature, humidity, and ventilation of the bedroom.

11. Ensuring that the bed is comfortable.

12. Using the bedroom exclusively for sleeping (avoiding things like watching TV, working on a computer, etc.).

13. Creating a "worry list" if something is bothering you.

relaxation techniques

Relaxation techniques provide us with excellent methods that can be practiced with awareness anytime at our discretion. These techniques are especially important when we are just beginning to experience stress. In this case, most of the negative consequences of stress can be counteracted even before they occur. In a French study, Bonnefond and colleagues (2001) found benefits of short napping at work, an idea that supports the utility of relaxation and application at American worksites.

Various techniques have been suggested to achieve relaxation. In this workbook the methods of *yogic breathing*, *progressive muscle relaxation*, *autogenic training*, and *visual imagery* will be described in detail. Step-by-step instructions have also been provided on the MP3 files available online for this text. Other techniques of relaxation, such as yoga, meditation, and biofeedback, are also introduced in this workbook. However, these methods require personal instruction and supervision by a qualified and experienced person. Thus, the actual techniques for these methods have not been completely elaborated upon. The reader is provided with appropriate resources for obtaining further assistance. See Box 3.1, Yoga and Meditation (page 59).

yogic breathing, or *pranayama*

All of us breathe. Breathing is a vital function for life. However, we seldom pay attention to how we breathe, which is an important aspect of life and needs to be understood. The process of breathing has received special emphasis in the system of yoga. As mentioned earlier, this process is known as *pranayama*. The purpose of this technique is not only to increase the vital capacity of the lungs but also to enhance the oxygenation capacity of the blood by the lungs. The oxygen from the air that we breathe in is carried by the hemoglobin in the blood to the various parts of the body, where it is used to release energy. If greater oxygen can be carried by the blood, then greater restoration of energy that has been lost in daily activities can be achieved. Therefore, the process of yogic breathing, or *pranayama*, is essential for achieving relaxation and managing stress. In simple terms, yogic breathing consists of three stages (Vasu, 1915):

○ *Puraka* (inhalation)

○ *Kumbhaka* (pausing or holding the breath)

○ *Rechaka* (exhalation)

BOX 3·1

Yoga and Meditation

Fundamentally, relaxation techniques owe their origin to Eastern cultures, particularly India. They are a part of the overall system of yoga that originated from the *Vedas*. The word *yoga* is derived from the Sanskrit root meaning "union," implying the joining or yoking of human consciousness to the Divine Being. According to *Webster's New World Dictionary* (1991), **yoga** is a mystic and ascetic Hindu discipline by which one seeks to achieve liberation from the material world and union with the supreme spirit or universal soul through intense concentration, deep **meditation**, and practices involving prescribed postures and controlled breathing. It is a complete system of physical, mental, social, and spiritual development of the human being. A contemporary description of yoga is "a systematic practice and implementation of mind and body in the living process of human beings to keep harmony within self, within society, and with nature" (Maharishi, 1986, 1987, 1989).

For generations this philosophy was passed on from the master teacher to the student. The first written records appeared around 200 b.c. in *Yogasutra* of Patanjali. It was known as *asthangayoga*, or the eightfold path of physical, psychological, and moral discipline, which if properly adhered to under the guidance of a qualified teacher, results in enhancement of purity and improved stress coping skills (Singh, 1983). This eightfold path of *asthangayoga* consists of the following:

1. *Yama:* Restraints or rules for living in society—for example, truthfulness, noninjury, and nonstealing

2. *Niyama:* Observances or rules for self—for example, contentment and cleanliness

3. *Asaana:* Physical exercises

4. *Pranayama:* Regulated breathing practice

5. *Pratihara:* Detaching the mind from senses

6. *Dharana:* Concentration on an object (internal or external)

7. *Dhyana:* Meditation

8. *Samadhi:* Deep meditation on the cosmic level

This process involves arousal of the *kundalini shakti*, or serpent power, believed to be located at the base of the human spine. As the practitioner practices the various techniques, this power rises through a series of centers or *chakras* corresponding to various endocrine glands. When this power reaches the highest center, *Sahasrara*, which is associated with the hypothalamus gland regulating the hormonal secretion of the endocrine glands, control over the hypothalamus results. In this way secretion of hormones from various endocrine glands can be regulated. This mechanism could possibly explain the important role that this method plays in coping with stress.

In the past, yoga was a strict and tedious process and was confined to only a select few. However, many teachers later modified the techniques and various paths emerged, such as *bhakti yoga*, the path of devotion; *gyana yoga*, the path of knowledge; *raja yoga*, the path of wisdom to self-realization and enlightenment; and *karma yoga*, the path of action. Various intermediary techniques like *hatha yoga*, *mudra yoga*, and *chakra yoga* have also gained popularity.

The system of yoga is in the process of developing as a science. Various simplified techniques of yoga have developed and gained popularity all over the world, particularly in the West. Examples of prevalent systems in the West include transcendental meditation (TM), *kriya yoga*, and simplified kundalini yoga (SKY).

Transcendental meditation (TM) was developed by Maharishi Mahesh Yogi, disciple of Brahmananda Saraswati, in 1957. In 1971 he founded the Maharishi International University in Fairfield, Iowa. In 1975 he established the International Capital of the Age of Enlightenment at Seelisberg in Switzerland, which has now been renamed Maharishi European Research University. TM is a simple, natural technique that can be learned by any person belonging to any age, education, occupation, or cultural background. It has to be practiced every day for 15 to 20 minutes and requires personal instruction by a qualified master who can gauge normal progress and take care of any adverse experiences if they arise. Centers teaching this technique are established all over the world, and the

(continued)

BOX **3·1**

Yoga and Meditation

process consists of the following seven steps (Kumar, 1993):

1. Introductory lecture—a vision of the possibilities through TM (60 minutes)

2. Preparatory lecture—the origin and mechanics of TM (60 minutes)

3. Personal interview with the teacher (15 minutes)

4. Personal instruction—learning the technique (60 minutes)

5. Verification and validation of experiences—verifying the correctness of the practice (90 minutes)

6. Understanding the mechanics of stabilizing the benefits of TM (90 minutes)

7. Understanding the mechanics of development of higher states of consciousness through TM (90 minutes)

Further information about learning transcendental mediation is available by visiting the Transcendental Meditation Program website at *www.tm.org*.

Kriya yoga became popular in the West due to the efforts of Paramhansa Yogananda, who founded the Yogoda Satsanga Society in India and the Self-Realization Fellowship in the United States. The word *kriya* is derived from the Sanskrit root *kri*, meaning "to do," "to act," and "to react." *Kriya yoga* involves a psychophysiological method by which human blood is decarbonated and recharged with oxygen. This extra oxygen is converted into life current to rejuvenate the central nervous system, lessen and prevent the decay of

tissues, and enhance evolution of the mind (Yogananda, 1946). Further information on this technique and system is available from Self-Realization Fellowship, *www.yogananda-srf.org*.

A better and more refined system is Yogiraj Vethathiri Maharishi's *simplified kundalini yoga* (SKY). Yogiraj Vethathiri Maharishi formed the World Community Service Center in 1958. This system was developed as a result of many years of extensive practice and research (Maharishi, 1986, 1987, 1989). It involves the arousal, awakening, and development of *kundalini shakti*, which lies dormant in most individuals at *mooladhara*, the base of the spine. The energy levels are raised to *agna chakra* and then to *sahasrara*. The important aspect of this system is *shanti yoga*, which helps keep control of the powerful awakened *kundalini shakti*. Other important aspects of this system include simplified physical exercises; introspection, or analysis of thoughts (as described in Chapter 6); and *kaya kalpa*, which is a system of exercises designed to improve upon health and longevity. Further information is available on the World Community Service Center website at *www.vethathiri.org*.

Other systems of meditation include (Naranjo & Omstein, 1971):

- *Soto Zen*, which involves focusing on external objects

- *Rinzai Zen*, in which the mind has to focus on koans (unanswerable, illogical riddles)

- *Zazen*, in which the mind focuses on subjective states of consciousness

- *Tibetan meditation*, in which the mind has to focus on geometric figures

The ratio of these three stages is 1:4:2—that is, one inhales the air for 4 seconds, then holds the air for 16 seconds, and then exhales the air over a period of 8 seconds. The purpose of yogic breathing is to achieve this kind of rhythmic breathing. We sometimes achieve this kind of breathing pattern when we are engrossed in some task with deep concentration, or some of us may be naturally gifted with this kind of pattern. This type of breathing pattern helps the body relax and conserve energy. It has been found to be useful in curing chronic

Reflect upon the following barriers that might be hindering your path to relaxing effectively.

▨ *Working Long Hours*. Some of us, in our quest to earn greater material wealth or for other reasons, may be working more than is normally required. As a result, we may have less time to relax.

▨ *Brooding*. Repetitive thinking of the same thoughts over and over again is brooding. It is often counterproductive and a barrier to relaxation.

▨ *Unchecked Imagination*. If we do not put a restriction on our imagination, then we may generate thousands of ideas in a short time that become barriers to relaxation.

▨ *Heavy Meals*. Eating more than required for maintaining your body function often results in indigestion. It also liberates greater energy. These factors hinder effective relaxation.

▨ *Inefficient Time Management*. Planning your time well is very important. If you do not provide yourself with adequate time for relaxation, you will not be able to relax properly.

▨ *Not Enough Faith in the Power of Relaxation*. It is essential for any method to be really effective that it command respect and faith from those utilizing it. Some of us do not have enough faith in the power of relaxation. This lack of faith colors our perspective and prevents us from getting complete relaxation.

muscle fatigue, migraine and tension headaches, and other stress-related disorders. **Worksheet 3.1**, on page 70, is based upon the traditional basic principles of yogic breathing, but has been slightly modified to make it feasible for modern times and give it universal applicability. Women, however, are advised not to follow this technique during the course of pregnancy and the postpartum period because it may cause unwanted pressure and/or hormonal changes that may affect the growing fetus.

Thoughts for Reflection 3.1, Barriers to Relaxation, above, will help you to reflect upon some of the barriers that may be hindering you from relaxing.

biofeedback

Biofeedback has been defined as the use of instrumentation to mirror psychological processes of which the individual is not normally aware and which may be brought under voluntary control (Brown, 1974; Fuller, 1977; Karlins & Andrews, 1972; Schwartz & Andrasik, 2005). The primary objective of biofeedback is monitoring and modifying the psychophysiological response that is obtained by enhancing awareness of internal states connected with deep levels of relaxation. Usually, information about internal vital functions such as blood pressure, heart rhythm, muscle tension, and so on is electronically recorded. This information is then explained to the participant, who is then encouraged to work gradually at modifying the responses by exerting greater relaxation. Gradually, the participant is able to gain greater modifying power of these internal functions that contribute to the reduction of stress. Biofeedback is normally administered with the help of a therapist. (Sessions usually last up to one hour depending upon discussions with the therapist.) The process involves three phases:

○ Measurement of the psychophysiological parameters

○ Conversion of these parameters into simple, understandable forms

○ Feedback of this information to the participant

Some of the instruments utilized in biofeedback laboratories are the *electromyograph* (EMG), which measures muscle tension and relaxation; *thermal units*, which measure skin-surface temperature; the *electroencephalograph* (EEG), which measures brain wave activity monitored from sensors placed on the scalp; and *galvanic skin response* (GSR) *units*, which measure sympathetic nervous system changes by recording the changes in sweat response on the skin's surface. Some conditions that are responsive to biofeedback include phobias, anxiety, hypertension, bruxism, asthma, headaches, insomnia, circulatory problems like Raynaud's disease, muscle spasms, and temporomandibular joint syndrome (Stoyva & Budzynski, 1993). The chief advantages of biofeedback practice are (Greenberg, 2010):

○ A greater control over the body and mind for the participant

○ A useful tool for psychologists to monitor bodily reactions to various stressors

○ An improvement in self-reliance of the participant in coping with stress

A simple form of biofeedback can be obtained with the help of biodots. *Biodots* are small, circular, microencapsulated cholesteric liquid crystals that measure a broad thermal range. In simple terms, they are miniature thermometers that measure skin temperature. Used as a very general indicator of skin temperature variance, they are designed to be triggered at a temperature higher than 87°F. Biodots are a versatile and economical tool for persons trained to interpret thermal responses. They are an ideal yet affordable device for an introductory example to persons unfamiliar with the most general biofeedback techniques. A biodot can be applied to almost any part of the body. However, the most ideal location is the gentle dip between the thumb and forefinger (Figure 3.1). This site provides the participant with a constant view of the biodot to monitor color change. It is necessary to remember that biodots are the simplest form of biofeedback, and therefore a great amount of trade-off has to be taken into account in terms of their accuracy. Biodots may not be able to provide accurate color change for many of us, especially for those of us who typically have cold hands. Room temperature also interferes with accurate measurement.

Biodots can be purchased from Biodot International (www.biodots.net/about). The various color changes that these biodots undergo are depicted in Table 3.1. For more information about biofeedback, access the Association for Applied Psychophysiology and Biofeedback (formerly the Biofeedback Society of America) website at www.aapb.org.

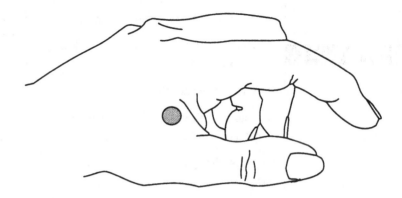

Figure 3.1 Site of Biodot Application

Table 3.1 COLOR CHANGES ON BIODOTS AND THEIR INTERPRETATIONS

Color	Temperature	Interpretation
Black	87.5° F	▪ Indicative of highly tense moment ▪ Normal initial color of the biodot
Amber	89.6° F	▪ Indicative of tense moment
Yellow	90.6° F	▪ Unsettled
Green	91.6° F	▪ Involved with the things going on around the person
Turquoise	92.6° F	▪ Starting to relax
Blue	93.6° F	▪ Calm
Violet	94.6° F	▪ Very relaxed

progressive muscle relaxation

Progressive muscle relaxation (PMR) was first described by Chicago physician Edmund Jacobson (1938, 1977). Jacobson designed this technique for hospital patients who were tense before surgery. He observed that these patients exhibited tenseness of small-muscle groups, such as the muscle groups located in the back or neck, and thus were unable to relax. Therefore, he taught these patients to first contract a set of muscles to experience tension and then gradually relax them. This process enabled individuals to discriminate between a relaxed and a tense state. It was repeated for all other muscle groups throughout the body.

The skeletal muscles in the body, which are arranged in various groups, number 1,030. All these muscles can be relaxed by PMR, one group of muscles at a time. This method has been found to be an excellent way to achieve relaxation of not only the skeletal muscles but also the mind and other internal organs. The primary feature of this method is the ability acquired by the practitioner to be able to selectively relax his or her muscle fibers on command at any time (McGuigan, 1993).

Jacobson spent over seven decades collecting data documenting the effectiveness of PMR in a scientific manner. This method has been shown to have application as a prophylactic method to reduce stress and tension. It also has applicability as a

Before going to bed every day, think …

▨ Did I work less, enough, or more? If less
or more, then contemplate why.

▨ Am I getting enough relaxation?

▨ Is there anything about my lifestyle that I
need to change?

Before beginning any new task or activity,
think …

▨ Is it worth all the effort?

▨ Is there any other way to do it better?

▨ Will it be beneficial to self, family, and
society?

▨ Can I do something else more beneficial
in the same time?

Before owning any new object, think …

▨ Do I really need it?

▨ Is it worth owning?

▨ What will be the consequences if I own
this object?

▨ What will be the consequences if I do
not own this object?

▨ Will it bring happiness and peace
to all?

Note: Based upon Eastern philosophy to obtain
relaxation and peace.

therapeutic measure. Its efficacy has been studied in nervous hypertension, acute insomnia with nervousness, anxiety neurosis, cardiac neurosis, chronic insomnia, cyclothymic depression, compulsive neurosis, hypochondria, fatigue states, nervous depression, and phobias. It also has been successfully applied to somatoform disorders such as convulsive tic, esophageal spasm, mucus colitis, chronic colitis, arterial hypertension, and tension headaches (McGuigan, 1993).

Bernstein and Carlson (1993) describe a shorter version of PMR known as abbreviated progressive relaxation training (APRT). Attempts to shorten the process of PMR were initiated by Joseph Wolpe (1958), whose method focused on relaxing several major muscle groups in seven sessions in contrast to Jacobson's program, which focused on a single muscle group for several sessions before moving on to the next. Paul (1966) further modified this shorter version and Bernstein and Borkovec formalized it (1973). We have, in this workbook, described a modification of all these methods that also includes some ideas from Eastern thought. You may now practice this method with the help of **Worksheet 3.2** (page 72).

Thoughts for Reflection 3.2, Think!, above, will help you to ponder appropriate modifications of some of your lifestyle behaviors that can provide you with greater relaxation and harmony in life.

autogenic training

Autogenic training (AT) owes its origin to the work of German neurologist Johannes Heinrich Schultz. He described it as a self-hypnotic procedure (Schultz, 1932). Autogenic therapy is a derivative of hypnosis and has been also described as "psychophysiological self-control therapy" (Pikoff, 1984).

Since its origin in Germany, it has remained quite popular in European countries and Japan. This technique became known in North America when one of Schultz's followers, Wolfgang Luthe, a physician, immigrated to Canada and translated much of this work into English. Ample evidence shows that it is a useful stress-reducing technique. It is also useful as a curative approach in dealing with anxiety and related disorders (Luthe, 1970; Stetter & Kupper, 2002).

The term *autogenic* is derived from the Greek words *autos*, meaning "self," and *genos*, meaning "origin." Therefore, in this technique, the self-regulation and self-healing powers of the mind are channeled in a positive manner. The practitioner of autogenic training concentrates on his or her body sensations in a passive manner without directly or volitionally bringing about any change (Linden, 1993). The key sensations on which the mind is focused include those of *heaviness* and *warmth*. Focusing on these sensations provides the body with a feeling of relaxation because these sensations are normally associated with the relaxation process. With the help of **Worksheet 3.3** (page 75), you can practice a slightly modified version of this technique that incorporates its key principles.

visual imagery

Visual imagery is mental visualization with the help of imagination. It is an important component of all relaxation techniques and is somewhat akin to dreaming. It has been used both in the East and in the West. It is based on the principle that whatever we think and imagine has a profound impact on our body. The key emphasis of visual imagery lies in enhancing an individual's innate capacity to attain and maintain health (Miller & Lueth, 1978). This technique can be used to accomplish effective results in almost all aspects of life. For example, in the training of athletes, visual imagery is used extensively. Regular visual imagery training makes it possible for athletes to mentally visualize beforehand various situations (such as performing in front of large crowds or winning an event) and techniques (such as swinging a bat or shooting baskets). Regular practice of visual imagery has been shown to improve performance, especially in tournaments and competitions.

Within the context of relaxation, imagining relaxing scenes and images is a very useful way to bring about relaxation. Visual imagery can also be used to overcome barriers that hinder effective relaxation. **Worksheet 3.4** (page 76) will help you practice visual imagery for relaxation.

Thoughts for Reflection 3.3, Autosuggestion (page 66) provides you with some ideas for autosuggestions or self-talk that can enhance the benefits of relaxation.

self-hypnosis

Franz Mesmer (1734–1815) is sometimes considered the father of hypnosis. He popularized hypnosis in the 18th century. Since then, hypnosis has been used for a variety of therapeutic and nontherapeutic applications. Hypnosis is the induction of a deeply relaxed state through suggestions accompanied by suspension of critical faculties. It has been used in therapeutic settings to modify unhealthy behaviors or relieve troubling symptoms. For example, in helping a patient lose weight, the hypnotist may give a suggestion that the person no longer likes being obese, that he will exercise, or that he will eat less. Hypnosis has also been found useful for relieving pain in advanced stages of cancers.

Visual imagery is similar to hypnosis in that the power of suggestion is used to achieve a deep state of relaxation (Vickers & Zollman, 1999). A major difference between visual imagery and hypnosis is that visual imagery is self-induced as opposed to hypnosis, which is induced by the hypnotist. Using another person to achieve relaxation makes one dependent on that person, and this process is thus less attractive and less practical. Another variant of visual imagery is *self-hypnosis*, in which, along with achieving relaxation, one also uses affirmations similar to

Autosuggestion, or talking with oneself, is a powerful means to develop self-confidence and build healthy lifestyles. Dr. Emile Coué, a French psychotherapist, was the first to come up with the best-known phrase for autosuggestion—"Day by day in every way, I am getting better and better" (Patel, 1993).

Reflect upon the following ideas for possible autosuggestions within the context of bringing relaxation in your life. After thinking through this list, you may wish to come up with a personal list of autosuggestions for yourself. These autosuggestions can be repeated to yourself during your free time, or routinely during morning and evening, or coupled with other relaxation methods.

- I am happy, healthy, and relaxed.

- I am in harmony with my surroundings.

- I work efficiently and sufficiently.

- I enjoy complete peace of mind.

- My sleep is sound, refreshing, and relaxing.

- My relationship with self and others is cordial.

- I stay calm and relaxed even in potentially tense situations.

- All the organs and organ systems in my body are working and relaxing optimally.

---

the suggestions used in hypnosis. *Affirmations* are positive and rational statements made by oneself to counter stressors and unpleasant thoughts. These affirmations are tailored and individualized.

In order to practice self-hypnosis you will first need to develop a set of affirmations. In **Worksheet 2.4** you identified things that cause you stress. You can develop a set of affirmations based on those stressors to use in your self-hypnosis practice. You can also use Thoughts for Reflection 3.3 to identify some autosuggestions that you would like to use. You can then use **Worksheet 3.4** (page 76) to relax. After you have reached a deep state of relaxation, you must focus on being aware of the present. Then, you can repeat to yourself the affirmations you have developed.

humor, stress, and relaxation

Humor is a word that has many meanings. Hippocrates identified the four humors: blood, phlegm, yellow bile, and black bile. According to Hippocrates, a balance between these four humors was essential for health. These humors correspond to the Latin meaning of the word, which is "liquid." Another meaning of the word *humor* refers to the comical or amusing aspect of a situation, person, or thing. We are interested in exploring the relationship of the latter meaning of humor with stress and relaxation.

Norman Cousins (1979) was perhaps among the first to give the low-down on the potential therapeutic effects of humor and laughter in his book *Anatomy of an Illness*. Humor has been found to be a moderator or a buffer in stress (Abel, 1998; Mauriello & McConathe, 2007). Humor perception involves the whole brain and serves to integrate and balance activity in both hemispheres (Wooten, 1996). Immunological research has shown that laughing lowers serum cortisol levels, increases the amount of activated T lymphocytes, increases the number and activity of natural killer cells, and increases the number of T cells that have helper/suppressor receptors (Berk, 1989a, 1989b). In other words, humor enhances the immune system that is suppressed by stress.

mindfulness meditation

A meditation technique derived from traditions of yoga and Buddhist meditation is mindfulness meditation. The technique has been popularized in the United States by Jon Kabat-Zinn, who developed the mindfulness-based stress reduction (MBSR) program that has been adopted by several hospitals around the country. Mindfulness meditation is an effective means for reducing stress and anxiety that accompanies daily life and chronic illness (Praissman, 2008). Studies have shown that mindfulness meditation is helpful in generalized anxiety disorder (Evans et al., 2008), chronic pain (Kabat-Zinn, Lipworth, & Burney, 1985), headache (Sun, Kuo, & Chiu, 2002), chronic low back pain (Morone, Greco, & Weiner, 2008), depression (de Zoysa, 2011), attention deficit hyperactivity disorder (Zylowska et al., 2008), and stress reduction in rheumatoid arthritis (Pradhan et al., 2007).

Mindfulness meditation entails "becoming aware" of your present. It is different from concentration, in which one focuses attention on one particular object. In mindfulness meditation one becomes aware of every aspect of experience. Sometimes a focus on breath is used to focus on the present moment, but other than that, no attempt is made to direct one's attention to any object. Mindfulness meditation can be done in any posture—sitting, lying down, or standing. In mindfulness meditation any activity done mindfully becomes a form of meditation, and it is possible to practice constantly while doing daily chores.

CHAPTER REVIEW

summary points

- ○ Relaxation is essential for normal functioning of all living beings. Relaxation techniques are the core of all stress management programs.

- ○ The natural process of relaxation is sleep. Sleep conserves and restores energy.

- ○ Sleep has two phases: rapid eye movement (REM) and non-rapid eye movement (non-REM). During the non-REM phase, the mind reaches subtler frequencies as recorded on an electroencephalograph (EEG).

- ○ Some techniques for relaxation are yoga; meditation; yogic breathing, or *pranayama;* progressive muscle relaxation (PMR); autogenic training (AT); and visual imagery.

- ○ Yoga is a systematic application of the mind and body to achieve overall harmony and peace.

- ○ Some systems of yoga popular in the West include transcendental meditation (TM), kriya yoga, and simplified kundalini yoga (SKY).

- ○ Biofeedback utilizes instruments to provide awareness about bodily functions that may then be brought under voluntary control.

- Progressive muscle relaxation (PMR) was first described by Edmund Jacobson. It is an effective means of achieving relaxation. PMR involves tensing and relaxing of muscles.

- Autogenic training was first described by J. H. Schultz and utilizes the self-regulation and self-healing processes of the mind to achieve relaxation.

- Visual imagery, or mental visualization with the help of imagination, is an important component of all relaxation procedures.

- Self-hypnosis is a variant of visual imagery that includes suggestive affirmations.

- Humor is a moderator or buffer for stress.

important terms defined

biofeedback: A method or set of methods that utilizes instruments to gauge physiological body functions that an individual is normally not conscious about and giving input from these measurements to the conscious mind in order to enhance greater volitional control over these functions.

meditation: A process of inner travel aimed at inducing peace by quieting the activity in the mind and fostering an experience of "being" rather than "doing."

pranayama: A method or set of techniques based on ancient yoga for increasing awareness and control on the unconscious activity of breathing, enhancing diaphragmatic activity, and enhancing inner energy levels. *See also* **yoga.**

progressive muscle relaxation: A relaxation method used to contract and then relax muscles of the arms, legs, face, neck, shoulders, and trunk.

relaxation technique: A method or a set of methods aimed at relieving bodily muscular strains and mental stress.

yoga: A Sanskrit word meaning "union." An ancient set of techniques aimed at inducing harmony between human and nature.

websites to explore

NATIONAL SLEEP FOUNDATION

www.sleepfoundation.org

This is the website of the National Sleep Foundation (NSF). Established in 1990 as an independent nonprofit organization, it is dedicated to improving public health and safety by achieving public understanding of sleep and sleep disorders and by supporting public education, sleep-related research, and advocacy.

- Explore this website to find out about the results from the national poll on sleep that this organization conducts. Are American adults sleeping enough? How often do Americans experience sleep disorders? Is drowsy driving a problem in America?

RELAXATION LINKS

http://stress.about.com

The website provides links to web resources dealing with various relaxation techniques and exercises, including imagery, meditation, progressive muscle relaxation, breathing techniques, and so on.

▧ Find a technique on the website that is not mentioned in this workbook and practice it.

THE OSHO WEBSITE

www.osho.com

This website describes the various teachings of Rajneesh, or Osho, a controversial Indian philosopher. The website introduces the teachings through audio files, video clips, and active meditation instructions.

▧ Explore this website; read, listen to, or watch a talk by this philosopher; and summarize your reaction in the form of a brief paper.

THE VETHATHIRI WEBSITE

www.vethathiri.edu.in

This website describes the life and teachings of an Indian saint and philosopher, Yogiraj Vethathiri Maharishi.

▧ Explore the website to read his teachings and prepare a paper comparing and contrasting his teachings with those of Osho or Maharishi Mahesh Yogi.

TRANSCENDENTAL MEDITATION

www.tm.org or
www.maharishi.org

Maharishi Mahesh Yogi is an Indian saint and philosopher who refined and introduced to the world the technique of transcendental meditation.

▧ Explore these websites to read about his life and views on various aspects. Discuss some things you like and dislike about this method. Have you learned any meditation techniques? Think about possible benefits of meditation.

Yogic Breathing, or Pranayama

You can practice yogic breathing at any time, but you should not have eaten 2 hours previously. The best time to perform this technique is early morning on an empty stomach or in the evening before supper. Pregnant women should *not* do this during the course of their pregnancy or immediate postpartum period. Complete this worksheet using the script below, or listen to track 2 on the MP3 files available online for this text.

A. BASIC BREATHING

Step 1. Sit down in a relaxed position. The ideal posture is squatting with the legs crossed. Place a watch in front of you.

Step 2. Inhale deeply and slowly. As you inhale, fill your lungs completely, starting from the lower section to the middle and proceeding to the upper section. Mentally record the time of completing the inhalation. For beginners this time could range anywhere from 4 to 16 seconds. With practice this time can be increased. Traditionally, there is no limit to the time; however, we recommend that you not exceed 20 seconds for the process of inhalation without supervision from an experienced practitioner.

Step 3. Hold your breath for a duration of four times the amount of time that you took to complete the inhalation.

Step 4. Exhale the air slowly in twice the amount of time you took to complete inhaling or half the time you took to hold your breath.

Step 5. Repeat Steps 2–4 five times over the first week. Then gradually increase the number of times over the next few months. We recommend that repetitions in one sitting not exceed 50, with no more than two sessions a day at that level unless supervised by an experienced practitioner.

B. BENDING BREATHING

Step 1. Kneel down or stand up straight.

Step 2. Inhale slowly and completely. First fill the lower section of the lungs, then the middle, and finally the upper section.

Step 3. While bending down from your original position, gradually exhale the air completely. You may take approximately the same amount of time that you took for inhaling.

Step 4. While rising up from your original position, gradually inhale and fill your lungs completely.

Step 5. Repeat Steps 2–4 five times the first week. Gradually increase your frequency over the next few months. We recommend a maximum of 20 repetitions per day.

C. ALTERNATIVE BREATHING

Step 1. Sit in a comfortable position.

Step 2. Close your right nostril with the thumb of your right hand.

Step 3. Inhale air slowly and completely through your left nostril.

Step 4. Exhale air slowly and completely through your left nostril.

Step 5. Repeat Steps 2–4 five times.

Step 6. Close your left nostril with the index and middle fingers of your right hand.

Step 7. Inhale air slowly and completely through your right nostril.

Step 8. Exhale air slowly and completely through your right nostril.

Step 9. Repeat Steps 6–8 five times.

Step 10. In this step you should practice alternative breathing. Close your right nostril with

Yogic Breathing, or Pranayama (*cont'd*)

your right thumb and inhale air slowly and completely through your left nostril. As soon as you complete inhalation, close your left nostril with the index and middle fingers of your right hand. Exhale air through the right nostril.

Step 11. Repeat Step 10 five times.

Step 12. Close your left nostril with the index and middle fingers of your right hand. Inhale air slowly and completely through your right nostril. As soon as you complete inhalation, close your right nostril with the thumb of your right hand. Exhale air through your left nostril.

Step 13. Repeat Step 12 five times.

FEEDBACK ON WORKSHEET 3.1

Yogic breathing is a practice-based technique that has to be done regularly. You may do it one or two times a day. You need not exceed the maximal frequency. This is a useful technique, which if practiced regularly, can modify the conventional "fight or flight" response to stress and reduce undue anxiety. Once you have mastered the yogic breathing technique, you can also easily practice it to relieve stress. All you need to do is sit down and perform yogic breathing whenever you are stressed. A couple of breaths taken in will rechannel the response and reduce the negative stimulation associated with stress.

Progressive Muscle Relaxation

The method of progressive muscle relaxation described here is a slight modification of the classical approach as advocated by Edmund Jacobson (1938, 1977). The original method takes a longer time, requires greater practice, and is slightly more tedious. This method is a simplification of the classical approach and also incorporates the relaxation component of physical exercises advocated in simplified kundalini yoga (SKY), as described earlier (Maharishi, 1987).

PREPARATION

▨ Seek out a relatively quiet, distraction-free environment, where the practice can be continued for 30 minutes without any interruptions.

▨ Avoid any unnecessary movements (getting up, fidgeting, etc.) during this process.

▨ This technique is best practiced in a lying-down supine position with arms placed alongside the body and eyes closed (Figure 3.2).

PRACTICE SESSION

You may want to record the following steps in your own voice on a tape recorder, or listen to track 3 on the MP3 files available online for this text. Some people prefer to just repeat the instructions mentally. This approach may require familiarity with these steps, which can be gained by reading them two or three times.

Step 1. Relaxation of the Arms (6 minutes)

▨ Clench the left fist.
▨ Feel the tightness in the muscles of the left hand.
▨ Now, let go.
▨ Feel the relaxation in the muscles of the left hand.

▨ Clench the right fist.
▨ Feel the tightness in the muscles of the right hand.
▨ Now, let go.
▨ Feel the relaxation in the muscles of the right hand.

▨ Clench both fists together.
▨ Feel the tightness in the muscles of both hands.
▨ Now, let go.
▨ Feel the relaxation in the muscles of both hands.

▨ Bend the left arm at the elbow.
▨ Feel the tightness in the muscles of the left arm.
▨ Now, let go.
▨ Feel the relaxation in the muscles of the left arm.

▨ Bend the right arm at the elbow.
▨ Feel the tightness in the muscles of the right arm.
▨ Now, let go.
▨ Feel the relaxation in the muscles of the right arm.

▨ Bend both arms at the elbow.
▨ Feel the tightness in the muscles of both arms.

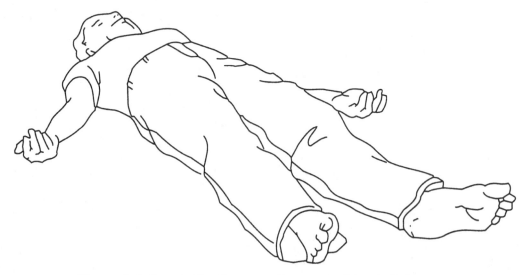

Figure 3.2 Position for Practicing Progressive Muscle Relaxation

Progressive Muscle Relaxation (*cont'd*)

- Now, let go.
- Feel the relaxation in the muscles of both arms.

Step 2. Relaxation of the Legs (7 minutes)

- Bend the left foot upward.
- Feel the tightness in the muscles of the left foot.
- Now, let go.
- Feel the relaxation in the muscles of the left foot.

- Bend the left foot downward.
- Feel the tightness in the muscles of the left foot.
- Now, let go.
- Feel the relaxation in the muscles of the left foot.

- Bend the right foot upward.
- Feel the tightness in the muscles of the right foot.
- Now, let go.
- Feel the relaxation in the muscles of the right foot.

- Bend the right foot downward.
- Feel the tightness in the muscles of the right foot.
- Now, let go.
- Feel the relaxation in the muscles of the right foot.

- Bend the left leg at the knee and tighten.
- Feel the tightness in the muscles of the left leg and thigh.
- Now, let go.
- Feel the relaxation in the muscles of the left leg and thigh.

- Bend the right leg at the knee and tighten.
- Feel the tightness in the muscles of the right leg and thigh.
- Now, let go.
- Feel the relaxation in the muscles of the right leg and thigh.

- Bend both legs at the knee and tighten.
- Feel the tightness in the muscles of both legs and thighs.
- Now, let go.
- Feel the relaxation in the muscles of both legs and thighs.

Step 3. Relaxation of the Face (5 minutes)

- Place wrinkles on the forehead by lifting the eyebrows.
- Feel the tightness in the muscles of the forehead.
- Now, let go.
- Feel the relaxation in the muscles of the forehead.

- Frown by drooping the eyebrows.
- Feel the tightness in the surrounding muscles.
- Now, let go.
- Feel the relaxation in the surrounding muscles.

- Close both eyes tightly shut.
- Feel the tightness in the surrounding muscles.
- Now, let go.
- Feel the relaxation in the surrounding muscles.

- Clench the jaw tightly.
- Feel the tightness in the surrounding muscles.
- Now, let go.
- Feel the relaxation in the surrounding muscles.

- Purse the lips tightly.
- Feel the tightness in the surrounding muscles.
- Now, let go.
- Feel the relaxation in the surrounding muscles.

Step 4. Relaxation of the Neck and Shoulders (6 minutes)

- Bend the neck gently forward.
- Feel the tightness in the muscles of the neck.
- Now, let go.
- Feel the relaxation in the muscles of the neck.

- Bend the neck gently backward.
- Feel the tightness in the muscles of the neck.
- Now, let go.
- Feel the relaxation in the muscles of the neck.

- Bend the neck gently to the right.
- Feel the tightness in the muscles of the neck.
- Now, let go.
- Feel the relaxation in the muscles of the neck.

(continued)

Progressive Muscle Relaxation (*cont'd*)

- Bend the neck gently to the left.
- Feel the tightness in the muscles of the neck.
- Now, let go.
- Feel the relaxation in the muscles of the neck.

- Shrug the left shoulder to touch the earlobe.
- Feel the tightness in the muscles of the left shoulder.
- Now, let go.
- Feel the relaxation in the muscles of the left shoulder.

- Shrug the right shoulder to touch the earlobe.
- Feel the tightness in the muscles of the right shoulder.
- Now, let go.
- Feel the relaxation in the muscles of the right shoulder.

Step 5. Relaxation of the Trunk (2 minutes)

- Inhale deeply to tighten the chest muscles.
- Feel the tightness in the muscles of the chest.
- Now, let go.
- Feel the relaxation in the muscles of the chest.

- Exhale with force to tighten the abdominal muscles.
- Feel the tightness in the muscles of the abdomen.

- Now, let go.
- Feel the relaxation in the muscles of the abdomen.

Step 6. Relaxation of the Whole Body (4 minutes)

Give yourself the following autosuggestions (see Thoughts for Reflection 3.3 on page 66).

- My feet are relaxed and healthy.
- My ankles are relaxed and healthy.
- My legs are relaxed and healthy.
- My knees are relaxed and healthy.
- My thighs are relaxed and healthy.
- My hips and pelvis are relaxed and healthy.
- My abdomen and parts within are relaxed and healthy.
- My chest and parts within are relaxed and healthy.
- My shoulders are relaxed and healthy.
- My arms are relaxed and healthy.
- My elbows are relaxed and healthy.
- My forearms are relaxed and healthy.
- My wrists are relaxed and healthy.
- My hands are relaxed and healthy.
- My neck is relaxed and healthy.
- My face is relaxed and healthy.
- My mind is relaxed and healthy.

FEEDBACK ON WORKSHEET 3.2

Progressive muscle relaxation is an excellent relaxation method with evidence to support its application as both prophylactic and therapeutic measures (Jacobson, 1938, 1977; McGuigan, 1993). The key to complete success lies in regular daily practice.

Autogenic Training

Autogenic training is a psychophysiological self-control technique for relaxation in which the person visualizes heaviness and warmth of arms and legs, followed by strength of heart, breathing, and visceral organs. The following steps are a slight modification of the conventional autogenic training method developed by Schultz (1932). If practiced regularly, this method can reduce stress and provide effective relaxation.

PREPARATION

Choose a quiet and comfortable place. You may practice this method either sitting or lying down. Choose a position in which you are comfortable. Close your eyes during this technique. You may either repeat the suggestions in the following steps mentally or listen to track 4 of the MP3 files available online for this text.

Step 1. Heaviness of the Arms (2 minutes)

- My right arm, forearm, and hand are getting heavy.
- I am feeling heaviness in my right arm, forearm, and hand.
- My left arm, forearm, and hand are getting heavy.
- I am feeling heaviness in my left arm, forearm, and hand.

Step 2. Heaviness of the Legs (2 minutes)

- My right thigh, leg, and foot are getting heavy.
- I am feeling heaviness in my right thigh, leg, and foot.
- My left thigh, leg, and foot are getting heavy.
- I am feeling heaviness in my left thigh, leg, and foot.

Step 3. Warmth in the Arms (2 minutes)

- My right arm, forearm, and hand are getting warm.
- I am feeling warmth in my right arm, forearm, and hand.
- My left arm, forearm, and hand are getting warm.
- I am feeling warmth in my left arm, forearm, and hand.

Step 4. Warmth in the Legs (2 minutes)

- My right thigh, leg, and foot are getting warm.
- I am feeling warmth in my right thigh, leg, and foot.
- My left thigh, leg, and foot are getting warm.
- I am feeling warmth in my left thigh, leg, and foot.

Step 5. Strength of the Heart (2 minutes)

- My heartbeats are regular and steady.
- My heart is strong and healthy.
- I am feeling strength in my heart.

Step 6. Strength of Breathing (2 minutes)

- My breathing is regular and steady.
- My lungs are strong and healthy.
- My respiratory tract is clear and healthy.
- I am feeling strength in my lungs and respiratory tract.

Step 7. Strength of All Visceral Organs (2 minutes)

- All my internal organs are healthy.
- I am feeling strength in all my internal organs.

Step 8. Coolness of the Forehead (2 minutes)

- My forehead is cool and relaxed.

Step 9. Finishing (1 minute)

- My body and mind are completely relaxed and rested.
- Gradually open your eyes and get up.

Visual Imagery

Find a quiet and comfortable place. Leave aside all your other activities for at least half an hour. If possible, the place should not have any sources of possible distraction, such as telephones, small children playing, and so on. You may choose to lie down or sit.

Complete this worksheet using the script below, or listen to track 5 on the MP3 files available online for this text.

▓ Close your eyes.

▓ Recollect the last time you were extremely happy. It may be that you were with someone; it may be that you had been somewhere; it may be that you got something. Whatever made you happy, mentally imagine that scene.

▓ Forget about everything else and just become engrossed in imagining that happy moment and scene.

▓ Remain with this feeling mentally for at least 10 minutes.

▓ Now imagine any event that you may not have experienced but that you believe will make you happy.

▓ Mentally enjoy the feeling of being in that event.

▓ Be with this feeling for at least 10 minutes.

▓ Now open your eyes and feel the relaxation and recharging of the body and mind that has taken place.

references and further readings

Abel, M. H. (1998). Interaction of humor and gender in moderating relationships between stress and outcomes. *The Journal of Psychology, 132,* 267–276.

Berk, L. (1989a). Neuroendocrine and stress hormone changes during mirthful laughter. *American Journal of Medical Science, 298,* 390–396.

Berk L. (1989b). Eustress of mirthful laughter modifies natural killer cell activity. *Clinical Research, 37,* 115.

Bernstein, D. A., & Borkovec, T. D. (1973). *Progressive relaxation training: A manual for the helping professions.* Champaign, IL: Research Press.

Bernstein, D. A., & Carlson, C. R. (1993). Progressive relaxation: Abbreviated methods. In P. M. Lehrer & R. L. Woolfolk (Eds.), *Principles and practice of stress management* (2nd ed.) (pp. 53–88). New York: Guilford Press.

Bixler, E. O., Kales, A., Soldatos, C. R., Kales, J. D., & Healey, S. (1979). Prevalence of sleep disorders in the Los Angeles metropolitan area. *American Journal of Psychiatry, 136,* 1257–1262.

Bonnefond, A., Muzet, A., Winter-Dill, A. S., Bailbenil, C., Bitouze, F., & Bonnean, A. (2001). Innovative working schedule: Introducing one short nap during the night shift. *Ergonomics, 44,* 937–945.

Brown, B. (1974). *New mind, new body, biofeedback: New directions for the mind.* New York: Harper & Row.

Centers for Disease Control and Prevention. (2011). Effect of short sleep duration on daily activities—United States, 2005–2008. *MMWR Morbidity and Mortality Weekly Report, 60*(8), 239–242.

Costa e Silva, J. A. (2006). Sleep disorders in psychiatry. *Metabolism, 55*(10, Suppl. 2), 540–544.

Cousins, N. (1979). *Anatomy of an illness.* New York: Norton.

Cumberbatch, C. G., Younger, N. O., Ferguson, T. S., McFarlane, S. R., Francis, D. K., Wilks, R. J., & Tulloch- Reid, M. K. (2011). Reported hours of sleep, diabetes prevalence and glucose control in Jamaican adults: Analysis from the Jamaica lifestyle survey 2007–2008. *International Journal of Endocrinology, 2011,* 716214.

de Zoysa, P. (2011). The use of Buddhist mindfulness meditation in psychotherapy: A case report from Sri Lanka. *Transcultural Psychiatry, 48*(5), 675–683.

Diagnostic and statistical manual of mental disorders (4th ed.) (DSM-IV). (1994). Washington, DC: American Psychiatric Association.

Evans, S., Ferrando, S., Findler, M., Stowell, C., Smart, C., & Halgin, D. (2008). Mindfulness-based cognitive therapy for generalized anxiety disorder. *Journal of Anxiety Disorders, 22*(4), 716–721.

Ford, D. E., & Kamerow, D. B. (1989). Epidemiology study of sleep disturbances and psychiatric disorders. An opportunity for prevention? *JAMA, 262,* 1479–1484.

Fuller, G. D. (1977). *Biofeedback: Methods and procedures in clinical practice.* San Francisco: Biofeedback Press.

Fuller, P. M., Gooley, J. J., & Saper, C. B. (2006). Neurobiology of the sleep-wake cycle: Sleep architecture, circadian regulation, and regulatory feedback. *Journal of Biological Rhythms, 21*(6), 482–493. doi: 10.1177/0748730406294627

Greenberg, J. S. (2010). *Comprehensive stress management* (12th ed). Boston: Brown/ McGraw-Hill.

Hall, M. H., Muldoon, M. F., Jennings, J. R., Buysse, D. J., Flory, J. D., & Manuck, S. B. (2008). Self-reported sleep duration is associated with the metabolic syndrome in midlife adults. *Sleep, 31*(5), 635–643.

Hirshkowitz, M. (2004). Normal human sleep: An overview. *Medical Clinics of North America, 88*(3), 551–565. doi:10.1016/j.mcna.2004.01.001

Hublin, C., Partinen, M., Koskenvuo, M., & Kaprio, J. (2007). Sleep and mortality: A population-based 22-year follow-up study. *Sleep, 30*(10), 1245–1253.

Jacobson, E. (1938). *Progressive relaxation* (2nd ed.). Chicago: University of Chicago Press.

Jacobson, E. (1977). The origins and developments of progressive relaxation. *Journal of Behavior Therapy and Experimental Psychiatry, 8,* 119–123.

Kabat-Zinn, J., Lipworth, L., & Burney, R. (1985). The clinical use of mindfulness meditation for the self-regulation of chronic pain. *Journal of Behavioral Medicine, 8*(2), 163–190.

Kalat, J. W. (1988). *Biological psychology* (3rd ed.). New York: Wadsworth.

Karlins, M., & Andrews, L. W. (1972). *Biofeedback: Turning on the powers of your mind.* New York: Lippincott.

Krauchi, K., & Wirz-Justice, A. (2001). Circadian clues to sleep onset mechanisms. *Neuropsychopharmacology, 25*(Suppl. 5), 592–596.

Kumar, C. S. C. (1993, August 29). What is TM? *The Week,* 10–15.

LeBow, O., Staner, L., Rivelli, S. K., Hoffmann, G., Pelc, I., & Linkowski, P. (2002). Correlations using the NREM-REM sleepcycle frequency support distinct regulation mechanisms for REM & NonRem sleep. *Journal of Applied Physiology, 93,* 141–146.

Linden, W. (1993). The autogenic training method of J. H. Schultz. In P. M. Lehrer & R. L. Woolfolk (Eds.), *Principles and practice of stress management* (2nd ed.) (pp. 53–88). New York: Guilford Press.

Luthe, W. (1970). *Autogenic therapy: Research and theory* (Vol. 4). New York: Grune & Stratton.

Maharishi, Y. V. (1986). *Karma yoga the holistic unity.* Madras, India: Vethathiri.

Maharishi, Y. V. (1987). *Simplified physical exercises.* Erode, India: Vethathiri.

Maharishi, Y. V. (1989). *Yoga for modern age.* Madras, India: Vethathiri.

Markov, D., & Goldman, M. (2006). Normal sleep and circadian rhythms: Neurobiologic mechanisms underlying sleep and wakefulness. *Psychiatric Clinics of North America, 29*(4), 841–853.

Mauriello, M., & McConathe, J. T. (2007). Relations of humor with perceptions of stress. *Psychological Reports, 101*(3, Pt. 2), 1057–1066.

McCoy, J.G., & Strecker, R.E. (2011). The cognitive cost of sleep lost. *Neurobiology of Learning & Memory, 96*(4), 564–582.

McGuigan, F. J. (1993). Progressive relaxation: Origins, principles, and clinical applications. In P. M. Lehrer & R. L. Woolfolk (Eds.), *Principles and practice of stress management* (2nd ed.) (pp. 17–52). New York: Guilford Press.

Miller, E. E., & Lueth, D. (1978). *Self imagery: Creating your own good health.* Berkeley, CA: Celestial Arts.

Mong, J. A., Baker, F. C., Mahoney, M. M., Paul, K. N., Schwartz, M. D., Semba, K., & Silver, R. (2011). Sleep, rhythms, and the endocrine brain: Influence of sex and gonadal hormones. *The Journal of Neuroscience, 31*(45),16107–16116.

Morone, N. E., Greco, C. M., & Weiner, D.K. (2008). Mindfulness meditation for the treatment of chronic law back pain in order adults: A randomized controlled pilot study. *Pain, 134*(3), 310–319.

Naranjo, C., & Ornstein, R. E. (1971). *On the psychology of meditation.* New York: Viking.

Patel, C. (1993). Yoga based therapy. In P. M. Lehrer & R. L. Woolfolk (Eds.), *Principles and practice of stress management* (2nd ed.) (pp. 89–137). New York: Guilford Press.

Paul, G. L. (1966). *Insight versus desensitization in psychotherapy.* Stanford, CA: Stanford University Press.

Pikoff, H. (1984). A critical review of autogenic training in America. *Clinical Psychology Review, 4,* 619–639.

Pradhan, E. K., Baumgarten, M., Langenberg, P., Handwerger, B., Gilpin, A. K., Magyari, T., et al. (2007). Effect of mindfulness-based stress reduction in rheumatoid arthritis patients. *Arthritis and Rheumatism, 57*(7), 1134–1142.

Praissman, S. (2008). Mindfulness-based stress reduction: A literature review and clinician's guide. *Journal of American Academy of Nurse Practitioners, 20*(4), 212–206.

Radecki, S. E., & Brunton, A. (1993). Management of insomnia in office-based practice. *Archives of Family Medicine, 2,* 1129–1134.

Schultz, J. H. (1932). *Das Autogene Training-Konzentrative Selbstentspannung.* Leipzig, Germany: Thieme.

Schultz, P. (2007). Biological clocks and the practice of psychiatry. *Dialogues in Clinical Neuroscience, 9*(3), 237–255.

Schwartz, M. S., & Andrasik, F. (2005). *Biofeedback: A practitioner's guide,* New York: Guilford Press.

Shapiro, C. M., & Flanigan, M. J. (1993). Function of sleep. *British Medical Journal, 306,* 383–385.

Singh, K. (1983). Hinduism. In *Religions of India.* New Delhi, India: Clarion Books.

Stepanski, E. J., & Wyatt, J. K. (2003). Use of sleep hygiene in the treatment of insomnia. *Sleep Medicine Reviews, 7*(3), 215–225.

Stetter, F., & Kupper, S. (2002). Autogenic training: A meta-analysis of clinical outcome studies. *Applied Psychophsiology and Biofeedback, 27*(1), 45–98.

Stoyva, J. M., & Budzynski, T. H. (1993). Biofeedback methods in the treatment of anxiety and stress disorders. In P. M. Lehrer & R. L. Woolfolk (Eds.), *Principles and practice of stress management* (2nd ed.) (pp. 263–300). New York: Guilford Press.

Sun, T. F., Kuo, C. C., & Chiu, N. M. (2002). Mindfulness meditation in the control of severe headache. *Chang Gung Medical Journal, 25*(8), 538–541.

Vasu, R. B. S. C. (1915). *An introduction to the yoga philosophy.* Allahabad, India: Panini Office.

Vickers, A., & Zollman, C. (1999). ABC of complementary medicine. Hypnosis and relaxation therapies. *British Medical Journal, 319,* 1346–1349.

Wolpe, J. (1958). *Psychotherapy by reciprocal inhibition.* Stanford, CA: Stanford University Press.

Wooten, P. (1996). Humor: an antidote for stress. *Holistic Nursing Practice, 10,* 49–57.

Yogananda, P. (1946). *Autobiography of a yogi.* Los Angeles: Self-Realization Fellowship.

Zhang, N., & Liu, H. T. (2008). Effects of sleep deprivation on cognitive functions. *Neuroscience Bulletin, 24*(1), 45–48.

Zylowska, L., Ackerman, D. L., Yang, M. H., Futrell, J. L., Horton, N. L., Hale, T. S., et al. (2008). Mindfulness meditation training in adults and adolescents with ADHD: A feasibility study. *Journal of Attention Disorders, 11*(6), 737–746.

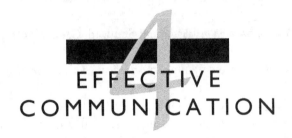

EFFECTIVE COMMUNICATION

"Think first before passing judgment."

what is communication?

We spend nearly 70 percent of our waking hours communicating—reading, writing, speaking, and listening (Robbins & Judge, 2012). If this communication becomes defective or faulty, it often leads to stress. Poor communication can be a source of anger, disagreement, distance in relationships, and misunderstandings which, if corrected, can result in stronger relations and happier future (Scott, 2011). Furthermore, this age of computer technology, email, chatrooms, and other web-based applications has added new complexities. Therefore, it is important for us to become effective communicators.

Before we proceed further, let's first define the term **communication**. One of the definitions that comes to mind is "transfer of meaning." *Is communication just transfer of meaning?* Perhaps it is more than just the transfer of meaning from one person to another. The important aspect of communication is the ability for the message to be understood: Unless the meaning is understood, communication will remain incomplete and ineffective. These two aspects—*transference* and *understanding*—are extremely complex in their dimensions. Since we communicate often, we seldom realize and appreciate the complexities involved.

Today, the English language has more than 600,000 words. According to linguists, an average educated adult uses about 2,000 of these words in daily conversation. The problem is that out of these words, 500 of the words most frequently used have more than 14,000 definitions (Burke, Hall, & Hawley, 1986). Each of us has a unique perspective in using and interpreting these words. More often than not, this multiplicity leads to problematic communication.

Furthermore, language is only a small tool that is used for communicating. A significant amount of communication involves nonverbal gestures, tone of voice, and so on. Complicating the matter further, we have several models of communication available to us. In our contemporary world, communication by email, Internet, and other technological advancements, although making the process faster, has also added several challenges (Box 4.1 on page 82).

the communication process

Berlo (1960) first described communication as a process. This model, known as the SMCR model (Sender, Message, Channel, Receiver), is one of the most popular (Figure 4.1 on page 83). The message to be conveyed passes between the sender (the source) and the receiver. The message is converted to a symbolic form (encoded) and is passed by way of some channel (medium) to the receiver who retranslates (decodes) the message initiated by the sender. In this way transference of meaning from one person to another results.

Let's try to understand what goes into each of these components. The *sender* initiates communication by encoding, or converting, a communication message to symbolic form. This process is influenced by the following factors:

○ *Knowledge* or information about the message—the factual components that may be correct or incorrect

○ *Skills* such as writing and speaking—the ability level of the sender to articulate the message

○ *Beliefs or convictions* that a phenomenon or object is true or real (Rokeach, 1970)—the impressions about the world

○ *Attitudes*, which are constant feelings directed toward an object (person, situation, or idea) and have an evaluative dimension (Green & Kreuter, 2005; Mucchielli, 1970)—beliefs with an evaluative component

○ *Values* or cultural intergenerational perspectives (Rokeach, 1970)—an enduring set of attitudes and beliefs that a mode of conduct is personally or socially preferable

The *message* is the actual physical product from the sender encoding it. For example, when we speak, the speech is the message; when we write, the writing is the message; when we gesture, the body movements are the message; and so on. The content of the message is important along with its elements, structure, and code and how it has been treated.

The medium through which a communication message travels is the *channel*. Any or all of the five senses—sight, hearing, smell, taste and touch—can be involved in the channel. Myers and Nance (1991) in *The Upset Book* have identified seven channels of communication:

1. Language—this is the "what" part of the message, the actual content or gist of the matter being conveyed.

2. Manner—this is how we express the message or say it vocally. The way in which a message is conveyed sometimes assumes greater importance than even the gist of what is said.

BOX **4.1**

Computer Technology Challenges for Stress Awareness

In present-day society, computer-aided communication has become a reality. Most of us have used email for communicating to family, friends, relatives, and professional contacts. We may have used the Internet for purchasing, getting information, chatting, and several other considerations. Some of us may have developed personal or professional web pages. Web-based chatting is becoming more and more common. These are all forms of communication that add new challenges to the process of communication. Some of the challenges that technology is posing are:

- *Less Time for Regular Communication.* Many of us have become so accustomed to new technology that we find less and less time for the traditional formal and informal means of communication. For many of us, this change creates a void in our normal day-to-day interactions and lessens our traditional social network. This reduction in conventional forms of networking also means reduction in conventional coping networks.

- *Speed of Communication.* Technology is becoming faster, and we are able to communicate at a much faster speed. Therefore, there is less time for thinking and proofreading as once was used in written communication. Oftentimes, this time pressure leads to miscommunication and creates stress for us and others.

- *Emerging and Fast-Changing Technology.* Technology changes so fast that by the time we feel comfortable with it, it is often obsolete. This unprecedented fast pace can be stressful.

- *Acronyms and Abbreviations.* People who are using computer-aided communication are finding and learning many new words, using language in a different way, learning abbreviations and acronyms, and using symbols to depict moods and feelings. For example, the acronym "lol" is used to convey the feeling "laughing out loud." Use of such newer forms of communication can add stress for the neophyte.

- *Junk Mail and Spamming.* Sometimes computer-aided communication is used by some people to vent their stress in the form of sending a lot of irrelevant junk mail to others (spamming). Besides stressing the computer network—it is stressful for all humans involved too!

- *Computer Worms and Viruses.* A worm is a program or algorithm that replicates itself over a computer network and usually performs malicious actions, such as using up the computer's resources and possibly shutting the system down. A virus is a program or piece of code that is loaded on one's computer unbeknownst to the user. Some people spitefully or unknowingly spread these viruses through the computer network and cause stress to others. For the person whose computer is infected, this can be a source of great stress.

While it may indeed be true that change is for the good and so are technological advancements—a little reflection on what these technological advancements and changes mean for us and our stress levels may give us a better insight into improving upon our communication and reducing stress levels in our lives.

3. Body language—this is how we express the message visually through our body movements. Use of gestures and actions adds flavor to the message.

4. Feelings or emotions—these are often inseparable from the communication process and are easily and automatically conveyed.

5. Symbolic communication—dress, hairstyle, and appearance, for example, are also important components that are consciously or unconsciously noticed.

6. Territory—this is personal space that includes both physiological and psychological dimensions.

7. Behavior—this includes intentional and not-so-intentional actions. The frequency, intensity, and duration of these actions can be documented.

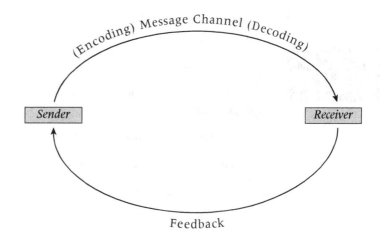

Figure 4.1 Berlo's SMCR Model of Communication

The *receiver* is the object to whom the message is directed. But before the message can be received, the symbols in it must be translated into a form that can be deciphered. This *decoding* is influenced by factors similar to those discussed earlier regarding encoding. The final link in the communication process is a *feedback loop*, which puts the message back into the system as a check against misunderstandings (Simonds, 1995). All of the seven channels are subject to possible distortion and can thereby contribute to the causes of stress.

You should now assess your ability to communicate through **Worksheet 4.1** (page 91). **Worksheet 4.2** (page 92) will help you identify your communication process in various situations and will provide feedback on ways to improve communication.

assertiveness

Another important aspect of communication is the ability to say no without feeling guilty. This is known as being *assertive*. Assertiveness has been defined as "expressing personal rights and feelings" (Lazarus, 1966; Wolpe, 1958). In another way it can be defined as expressing oneself, satisfying one's personal needs, feeling good about this, and not hurting others in the process (Greenberg, 2010). **Worksheet 4.3** (page 94), Assessing Assertive Behavior, will help you gain insight into **passive**, **assertive**, and **aggressive behaviors** when communicating with others.

Research shows that nearly everybody can be assertive in some situations, whereas in others the same person will be ineffectual. The goal is to increase the number and variety of situations in which assertive behavior is possible. Assertiveness decreases the events in which a passive behavior or a hostile blowup occurs.

Assertiveness is *not* the same as aggressiveness. One can differentiate between the two by asking three simple questions:

1. Am I violating someone else's rights?

2. Do others react to me by feeling angry or upset?

3. Do I intend to be malicious, or do I intend to be fair to all concerned?

1. You have the right to decide upon your behavior, thoughts, and emotions and to take responsibility for their initiation and consequences.

2. You have the right to offer no reasons or excuses for your behavior.

3. You have the right to judge if you are responsible for finding solutions to other people's problems.

4. You have the right to change your mind.

5. You have the right to make mistakes—and be responsible for them.

6. You have the right to say, "I don't know."

7. You have the right to be independent of the goodwill behavior of others before coping with them.

8. You have the right to be illogical in making decisions.

9. You have the right to say, "I don't understand."

10. You have the right to say, "I don't care."

Note: From *When I say no, I feel guilty* by Manuel J. Smith. Copyright 1975 by Manuel J. Smith. Used by permission of Doubleday, a division of Bantam Doubleday Dell Publishing Group, Inc.

Aggressiveness means seeking to dominate or to get your own way at the expense of others. This tendency should be curbed as far as possible and replaced with assertiveness. See Thoughts for Reflection 4.1, A Bill of Assertive Rights, above. Practice to be more assertive using the steps in **Worksheet 4.4** (page 96).

Worksheets 4.3 and **4.4** will provide you with an insight as to whether or not you are assertive. Some characteristics of an assertive person include:

○ Direct eye contact

○ Appropriate use of hand movements

○ Firm posture

○ Steady utilization of voice

○ Use of "I" statements

○ Speaking in short sentences

○ Feedback pauses

A person exhibiting assertiveness always uses direct eye contact by looking the other person in the eye while communicating. However, one has to remember that in some cultures direct eye contact is not encouraged. Therefore, absence of direct eye contact should not lead one to conclude absence of assertiveness. An assertive person utilizes appropriate hand movements while communicating, being careful not to cause discomfort or invade the other person's space. An assertive person engages in a firm posture, not too stiff, yet not too relaxed, which maintains an appropriate distance in which both parties are comfortable. An assertive person uses a steady, consistent voice, keeping emotion to a minimum. One of the key characteristics of an assertive person is the use of "I" statements, which demonstrates that an assertive person owns his or her behavior and is responsible for any consequence thereof.

Broken Record. A systematic communication skill in which we are persistent and keep saying what we want over and over without getting angry, irritated, or loud. By practicing to speak like a broken record, we learn to be persistent, stick to the point of discussion, and continue to say what we want. This technique helps us ignore all side issues brought up by the other party.

Workable Compromise. A technique to use with an equally assertive person to work out a compromise. A workable compromise is one in which our self-respect is not in question.

Free Information. A listening skill in which we evaluate and then follow up on the free information that people offer about themselves. It accomplishes two things. It makes it easier for us to converse comfortably with people, and it is assertively prompting others to speak easily and freely with us.

Self-Disclosure. A technique we use to assertively disclose information about ourselves. How we think, feel, and react to the other person's free information permits social communication to flow both ways. It goes hand in hand with free information, because to elicit more information, we must be willing to self-disclose.

Fogging. A response to assertively cope with manipulative criticism of others in which we do not deny any of the criticism, we do not get defensive, and we do not attack with criticism of our own. We set up a fog bank. It is persistent. It cannot be clearly seen through. It offers no resistance to penetration. It does not fight back and has no hard striking surfaces. Fogging permits us to cope by offering no resistance or hard psychological striking surfaces to critical statements thrown at us.

Negative Assertion. A technique in which we cope with criticism or with our errors and faults by openly acknowledging them. This technique is to be used only in social conflicts and not physical or legal ones.

Negative Inquire. An assertive, nondefensive response that is noncritical of the other person and prompts that person to make further inquiry to examine his or her own structure of right and wrong, which he or she is using in certain situations. For example, "I don't understand. What makes you think educators are stupid?"

Note: From *Stress stoppers: Managing stress effectively* (p. 25) by P. R. Kovacek, 1981, Detroit: Henry Ford Hospital.

An assertive person uses short sentences expressing clarity and brevity in thought. Finally, an assertive person often pauses to obtain feedback from others, which is vital for effective communication. Thoughts for Reflection 4.2, above, provides some ideas for becoming assertive, and Thoughts for Reflection 4.3 (page 86) describes nine types of assertive responses.

Another important aspect of communication is the ability to listen. It is human nature to prefer being the sender more often than the receiver. We have to remember that listening is more important for us to be effective (Covey, 1990). We will be discussing this aspect in depth in the next chapter when we talk about dealing with an angry person.

behavioral styles

Now that we have practiced assertiveness, let's focus our attention on another important aspect of communication—how we behave. All of us have developed certain behavioral patterns—distinct ways of thinking, feeling, and acting.

1. *Assertive Talk.* Do not let others take advantage of you. Expect to be treated with fairness and justice. Examples: "I was here first," "Please turn down the radio," "I've been waiting here for half an hour," "This steak is well-done, and I ordered it medium-rare."

2. *Feeling Talk.* Express your likes and dislikes spontaneously. Be open and frank about your feelings. Do not bottle up emotions, but don't let emotions control you. Examples: "What a marvelous shirt!" "How great you look!" "I hate this cold," "I'm tired as hell," "Since you ask, I do prefer you in another type of outfit."

3. *Greeting Talk.* Be outgoing and friendly with people whom you would like to know better. Do not avoid people because of shyness, or because you do not know what to say. Smile brightly at people. Look and sound pleased to see them. Examples: "Hi, how are you?" "Hello, I haven't seen you in months," "What are you doing with yourself these days?" "How do you like working at _____ ?" "Taking any good courses?"

4. *Disagreeing Passively and Actively.* When you disagree with someone, do not feign agreement for the sake of "keeping the peace" by smiling, nodding, or paying close attention. Change the topic. Look away. Disagree actively when you are sure of your ground. Use fogging with manipulative criticizers.

5. *Asking Why.* When you are asked to do something that does not sound reasonable or enjoyable by a person in power or authority, ask why you should do it. You are an adult and should not accept authority alone. Ask for reasonable explanations from teachers, relatives, and other authority figures. Have it understood that you will live up to voluntary commitments and be open to reasonable suggestions, but that you cannot comply with unreasonable orders.

6. *Talking About Oneself.* When you have done something worthwhile or interesting, let others know about it. Let people know how you feel about things. Relate your experiences. Do not monopolize conversations, but do not be afraid to bring them around to yourself when it is appropriate.

7. *Agreeing with Compliments.* Do not depreciate yourself or become flustered when someone compliments you with sincerity. At the very least, offer an equally sincere "Thank you." Or reward the complimenter by saying, "That's an awfully nice thing to say. I appreciate it."

8. *Avoiding Justification of Opinions.* Be reasonable in discussions, but when someone goes out of his or her way to dominate a social interaction by taking issue with any comments you offer, use a technique such as broken record.

9. *Looking People in the Eye.* Do not avoid the gaze of others. When you argue, express an opinion, or greet a person, look him or her directly in the eye.

Note: Adapted from Behavior research & therapy. II, S. A. Rathus, "Instigation of assertive behavior through video tape mediated assertive models and directed practice," pp. 57–65. Copyright 1973, with kind permission from Elsevier Science Ltd., The Boulevard, Langford Lane, Kidlington, OX5 1GB, UK.

The central core of these patterns tends to remain stable because it reflects our individual identities. However, the demands of the world around us (personal, family, school, and work) often require different responses that evolve into a consistent behavioral style (Carlson Learning Company, 1994). One of the tools to explain behavioral styles is the Personal Profile System® developed by Carlson

Learning Company of Minneapolis, Minnesota. This profile presents a plan to help us understand ourselves and others in our social or work environment.

The Personal Profile System (PPS) is a self-administered, self-development instrument. The profile was originally developed by John Geier (based upon extensive study of behavioral tendencies) and subsequently refined by Michael O'Connor (Carlson Learning Company, 1994). The Personal Profile System also utilizes the work of William Moulton Marston. He theorized that human behavior could be studied on a two-axis model according to a person's actions in a favorable or an antagonistic environment (Marston, 1979).

The focus of this instrument is to understand oneself so that one can understand others and place oneself in an environment that is conducive to success (Kaufman & O'Connor, 1992). This instrument measures four dimensions of behavioral responses, or DiSC (Carlson Learning Company, 1994):

○ **Dominance** (D): Emphasis is on shaping the environment by overcoming opposition to accomplish results.

○ **Influence** (i): Emphasis is on shaping the environment by influencing or persuading others.

○ **Steadiness** (S): Emphasis is on cooperation with others to carry out the task.

○ **Conscientiousness** (C): Emphasis is on a cautious, tentative response designed to reduce antagonistic factors in an unfavorable environment.

The behavioral dimensions can be divided into two categories—process or product orientation. Persons with predominantly Dominance or Influence tendencies are process oriented. They want to shape the environment according to their particular view. These are individuals who continually test and push the limits set by the group or organization. Those people with the Steadiness and Conscientiousness tendencies are product oriented. They focus on the how and the why. These people may at times need encouragement to reset limits.

For example, people with *dominance* tendencies have the results they want well in mind. Their messages are designed to stimulate and prod others to untested action. They are attentive to communication that will speed the action. Questions about the "correct" action are shrugged away. These individuals feel they can change the course of action (Performax Systems International, 1986).

People with *influence* tendencies also want to shape and mold events and have an active voice. Their messages are designed to stimulate and prod others to action by working with and through people. They are interested in people and like to make people feel good about themselves. They are particularly attentive to the personal needs of others and search for ways to meet those needs. Messages about how to actually accomplish a task are often deemed unimportant; these stimuli are at the far range of their attention span.

Persons with *steadiness* tendencies are interested in the how and when—a product orientation. They send messages that reflect their interest in maintaining a stability within themselves and the situation—between the old and the new. Messages that urge action before knowing how to do things fall on deaf ears.

Individuals with *conscientiousness* (to their own standards) tendencies reflect their product orientation when they send messages that ask the reasons for the change. "Why?" is a favorite question. They have concern for doing it "accurately." They are receptive to messages that reassure them they are doing it correctly. Messages that ignore this need tend to go unheeded.

BOX 4·2

Some Interesting Concepts in Communication and Their Relationship with Stress

The field of communication, like all fields, has some interesting and unique concepts. In this box, we discuss some concepts in communication and their relationship with stress. Some terms include *proxemics, metamessages, metacommunication,* and *paralanguage.*

Proxemics: Proxemics is an anthropological term that refers to the measurable distance between people when they interact. Each person has an *intimate space* for embracing, touching, or whispering with a radius of approximately 1.5 feet, a *personal space* for interactions among friends with a radius of approximately 4 feet, a *social space* for interactions among acquaintains with a radius of approximately 12 feet, and a *public space* for public speaking with a radius of approximately 25 feet. Different cultures have different standards of these spaces. If these standards are altered, it can produce stress. We need to be cognizant of the space that people find comfortable and plan communication accordingly.

Metamessages: Metamessages refer to the different meanings that come from messages because of various assumptions, implications, and interpretations. For example, someone says "How are you?" and you interpret whether it is a greeting or a genuine inquiry about your health. These two different interpretations make it a metamessage. Incorrect interpretation of

metamessages can lead to stress. Acknowledging and responding to metamessages is often more important than dealing with the literal meaning of the messages. We need to be careful when using and interpreting metamessages.

Metacommunication: Metacommunication is a form of communication that means different things at different levels. The word "meta" means *in addition to.* Therefore, metacommunication means implying more in addition to the manifest "content" of what is said. For example, some people are fond of saying "Trust me," when oftentimes the phrase conveys the exact opposite of its literal meaning. Use of metacommunication can potentially produce stress and must be avoided as far as possible. We must aim at keeping communication as simple as possible.

Paralanguage: Paralanguage pertains to nonverbal aspects of communication that either modify the meaning of what is said or convey emotion to what is being said. Paralanguage includes body language, tone of speech, pitch of speech, and volume of speech. Oftentimes paralanguage is conveyed unconsciously and has the potential to add stress in communication. We should attempt to become consciously aware of our paralanguage so that communication can become clearer and there is reduced potential for stress.

how the personal profile contributes to stress reduction

Box 4.2 above discusses some interesting concepts in communication and their relationship with stress. The Personal Profile System also provides considerable information about the way people respond to stress. This information can be effectively used to understand and help reduce stress. As noted in Chapters 1 and 2, the stress response consists of two components: "fight" or "flight." Hans Selye (1956) refined this concept into four distinct responses that correspond to our four primary behavioral tendencies:

○ *Fight.* The "high D" people will tend to use the fight response. They will attempt to destroy the impact of the stress or eliminate its cause. The fighting may be verbal or physical.

○ *Flight.* The "high i" people will tend to use the flight response. They will attempt to flee from the situation. If physical flight is not possible, they will attempt to flee emotionally by changing the subject or ignoring the issue. If the stress continues, they may become emotionally abusive.

○ *Tolerate.* The "high S" people will tend to use the tolerate response, which is really a subtle form of flight. They will not attempt to fight or flee; however, they will tend to shut down. They will remain in the situation with apparent calmness; however, they may become dysfunctional, not knowing what to do.

○ *Avoid.* The "high C" people will tend to use the avoid response, which is a subtle form of fight. They will not attempt to fight or flee; however, they will tend to withdraw in order to avoid conflict. They may in fact use the time as an opportunity to carefully plan their next move.

According to Kaufman and O'Connor (1992), if the level of stress becomes even more severe, individuals will tend to move step by step through the stress responses associated with behavioral styles more directive than their own. That is, a "high i" individual will first move from the flight response to the tolerate response characteristic of the "high S" individual. This individual will then move from the "tolerate" response to the "avoid" response, then to the "fight" response characteristic of the "high D." A "high S" individual will move through the "avoid" response to the "fight" response. A "high C" individual will move to the "fight" response. The "fight" response is the ultimate survival-level response. We will all resort to that behavior if the level of stress is high enough.

For further information and training on the Personal Profile System, visit www.discprofile.com. The PPS is also available online at www.inscapepublishing.com.

CHAPTER REVIEW

summary points

○ We spend approximately two-thirds of our waking hours communicating.

○ Faulty communication is at the root of most stress.

○ Berlo describes a popular model of communication, known as the SMCR (Sender, Message, Channel, Receiver) Model.

○ An important aspect of communication is assertiveness or the ability to say no without feeling guilty.

○ Being assertive produces the least amount of stress, whereas being passive or aggressive is more stressful.

○ Assertiveness is an acquired quality that everyone can develop.

○ Some techniques for becoming assertive include sounding like a broken record, compromising, providing free information, self-disclosure, fogging, negative assertion, and negative inquiry.

○ How we behave impacts how effectively we communicate.

○ The Personal Profile System is a tool to assess our behavioral styles. The Profile describes four responses: Dominance (D), Influence (i), Steadiness (S), and Conscientiousness (C).

important terms defined

aggressive behavior: A way of behaving in which the person tries to express his or her rights and feelings by dominating and usually getting his or her way at the expense of others. It involves covert or overt emotional aggravation.

assertive behavior: A way of functioning in which a person can express his or her rights and feelings without hurting anyone. It does not lead to emotional fluctuations.

communication: The process of transferring ideas, concepts, or notions from one person (sender or source) to another person or persons (receivers) through use of a symbolic form (message) sent via a channel (medium).

passive behavior: A way of functioning in which the person tries to avoid any expression of his or her rights or feelings at a given time.

websites to explore

DESIGNED THINKING

www.designedthinking.com/

This is the website of a commercial company that conducts workshops on communication techniques for reducing stress.

▦ Explore the website and find out about neurolinguistic programming (NLP) techniques. Write a brief summary paper.

DISC PROFILE

www.discprofile.com/

This website provides more information about the Personal Profile System.

▦ Read more about the system. The actual instrument for profiling can be ordered from this website.

EFFECTIVE COMMUNICATION

www.health.umd.edu/fsap/communication.html

This website from the University of Maryland provides excellent tips on improving communication for reducing stress.

▦ Read the information from this website and summarize your reaction in a brief paper about how you can make your point in an effective manner.

INTERPERSONAL COMMUNICATION ARTICLES

www.expressyourselftosuccess.com/tag/interpersonal-communication-articles/

This website presents several interesting articles on interpersonal communication and stress.

▦ Read and summarize one article in a brief paper.

4.1

1. 3   11. 2
2. 4   12. 4
3. 3   13. 4
4. 5   14. 2
5. 2   15. 3
6. 2   16. 4
7. 3   17. 5
8. 3   18. 5
9. 4   19. 3
10. 2   20. 4

Communication Assessment

This worksheet is a self-assessment tool that will enhance your awareness of various attributes of effective communication. There are no right or wrong answers. It can also be used for gathering feedback from others about you as a communicator. So, you can ask your spouse, a family member, friend, colleague, or someone who knows you to fill out this worksheet for you.

How would you rate yourself (or the person whom you are assessing) on the following items?

5 = excellent	2 = poor
4 = very good	1 = very poor
3 = satisfactory	

While communicating ...	Rating Scale				
1. I am concise and to the point.	5	4	3	2	1
2. I express myself clearly.	5	4	3	2	1
3. I modulate the tone of my voice to convey precise meaning.	5	4	3	2	1
4. I use appropriate body gestures and facial expressions.	5	4	3	2	1
5. I am forceful and definite rather than hesitant and apologetic.	5	4	3	2	1
6. I summarize the key points.	5	4	3	2	1
7. I do not talk in roundabout ways.	5	4	3	2	1
8. I am specific and give examples to make my points clear.	5	4	3	2	1
9. I let others know in unambiguous terms when I do not understand them.	5	4	3	2	1
10. I often ask others if they have understood me.	5	4	3	2	1
11. I help others participate in the discussion.	5	4	3	2	1
12. I listen actively.	5	4	3	2	1
13. I keep my feelings under check.	5	4	3	2	1
14. I do not react to the feelings of others.	5	4	3	2	1
15. I listen to understand rather than prepare for the next remark.	5	4	3	2	1
16. I avoid using jargon and use simple language.	5	4	3	2	1
17. I give equal respect to others as communicators.	5	4	3	2	1
18. I try to see the other person's point of view.	5	4	3	2	1
19. I do not divert myself while communicating.	5	4	3	2	1
20. I am able to withstand silence.	5	4	3	2	1

FEEDBACK ON WORKSHEET 4.1

Having rated yourself and also having elicited feedback from others, you will now be quite clear about your communication style strengths and limitations. Try to build further on your strengths (categories in which you have rated excellent and very good). Also try to overcome your limitations (categories in which you have rated yourself or have been rated as satisfactory, poor, or very poor).

Communication in Various Situations

Circle the answer that best describes what you would
do in each situation.

1. I have an important appointment in the next half
   hour and my best friend arrives. I would …
   a. ask my spouse to handle the situation and leave
      from the back door.
   b. exchange pleasantries and excuse myself politely.
   c. cancel the appointment.
   d. hurriedly leave.

2. I am working in a middle management position.
   The head of the organization invites me to lunch.
   When I return, I sense that my department head is
   curious. I would …
   a. ignore him or her.
   b. give a detailed description.
   c. mention the meeting casually—as though
      nothing has happened.
   d. fabricate a story.

3. My significant other is not able to keep a date with
   me. I would …
   a. act as if nothing has happened.
   b. ask him or her the reason.
   c. wait for his or her explanation.
   d. walk out on him or her.

4. My significant other tells me a juicy story about
   the neighbor's daughter that he or she has heard
   from somewhere. I would say …
   a. "I don't want to hear any of this."
   b. "I am not interested."
   c. "What happened next?"
   d. "How does it concern us?"

5. I have to stay late at the office completing pending
   work. I return home and am tired. My significant other
   inquires the reason for my coming in late. I would …
   a. tell him or her to mind his or her own business.
   b. explain the reason clearly.
   c. ignore him or her.
   d. change the topic of conversation.

6. In a staff meeting, my supervisor makes an inaccu-
   rate statement. I would …
   a. correct my supervisor on the spot.
   b. correct my supervisor later away from the meeting.

   c. ask a clarifying question at the meeting and
      discuss the matter later.
   d. tell other staff members how foolish my
      supervisor is.

7. I am at a party, and someone introduces me to
   a person of different ethnic orientation. After
   initiating conversation, I am unable to understand
   the other person. I would …
   a. politely excuse myself.
   b. ask the person for repeated clarifications.
   c. nod in agreement.
   d. form an opinion about his/her poor
      communication skills.

8. A friend calls me on the phone and invites me
   to a sports event. I have made other plans with
   another person but would very much like to go. I
   would …
   a. call my other friend and cancel the appointment
      so I can go to the sports event.
   b. ask my friend if the other person can come
      along to the sports event.
   c. persuade my friend to cancel going to the
      sports event and join me.
   d. cancel both engagements and stay at home.

9. I enter a meeting and find that all the members
   have burst into laughter. I would …
   a. assume that they are laughing at me and leave
      the meeting.
   b. assume that they are laughing at me and speak
      against their inappropriate behavior.
   c. laugh with them and later ask the reason for
      laughing.
   d. sit quietly and ask nothing.

10. I give my teenage son or daughter a specific time
    to be home. He or she openly defies my directive
    by coming home very late. I would …
    a. reprimand him or her and decide not to talk
       about it again.
    b. discuss the matter openly the next day.
    c. blame my spouse for spoiling the teenager.
    d. call up the other parents and complain.

FEEDBACK ON WORKSHEET 4.2

Responses that would help prevent undue stress in your life because of improper communication are as follows:

1. b This response would prevent any miscommunication and misunderstanding from occurring.

2. b You owe your loyalty to your immediate supervisor. If you fabricate, ignore, or do not tell enough, you will sow the seeds of mistrust.

3. b An open discussion would help you understand his or her problem.

4. d You need to avoid gossip that floats around unless it concerns you, and then try to find out the facts. In this way miscommunication and associated problems can be avoided.

5. b This response would prevent any miscommunication and misunderstanding.

6. c Asking a clarification question at the time of the discussion will help your supervisor correct himself or herself if he or she has made the statement out of oversight. If not, discussion at a later time will help clarify your point of view without embarrassing your supervisor.

7. b Repeated clarifications will help you understand what the other person is trying to communicate.

8. b Accomplishing your goals without hurting the feelings of others is a part of assertiveness and effective communication. Be upfront about your position.

9. c Laughing with people, even if you are being laughed at, will reduce undue discomfort for you. Soliciting clarification later on will help you understand the actual reason.

10. b An open discussion about the matter will help you both clarify your viewpoints and reach mutual understanding.

This worksheet should help you appreciate the importance of straightforwardness and assertiveness in your communication with others in order to reduce stress.

Assessing Assertive Behavior

To determine your general pattern of behavior, indicate how characteristic of you each of the following statements is by using the following code:

+3 = very characteristic of me, extremely descriptive
+2 = rather characteristic of me, quite descriptive
+1 = somewhat characteristic of me, slightly descriptive
−1 = somewhat uncharacteristic of me, slightly nondescriptive
−2 = rather uncharacteristic of me, quite nondescriptive
−3 = very uncharacteristic of me, extremely nondescriptive

_____ 1. Most people seem to be more aggressive and assertive than I am.

_____ 2. I have hesitated to make or accept dates because of shyness.

_____ 3. When the food served at a restaurant is not done to my satisfaction, I complain about it to the waiter or waitress.

_____ 4. I am careful to avoid hurting other people's feelings, even when I feel that I have been injured.

_____ 5. If a salesperson has gone to considerable trouble to show me merchandise that is not quite suitable, I have a difficult time in saying no.

_____ 6. When I am asked to do something, I insist upon knowing why.

_____ 7. There are times when I look for a good, vigorous argument.

_____ 8. I strive to get ahead of others in my position.

_____ 9. To be honest, people often take advantage of me.

_____ 10. I enjoy starting conversations with new acquaintances and strangers.

_____ 11. I often don't know what to say to people to whom I am sexually attracted.

_____ 12. I will hesitate to make phone calls to business establishments and institutions.

_____ 13. I prefer to apply for a job or admission to a college by writing letters rather than by going through personal interviews.

_____ 14. I find it embarrassing to return merchandise.

_____ 15. If a close and respected relative were annoying me, I would smother my feelings rather than express my annoyance.

_____ 16. I have avoided asking questions for fear of sounding stupid.

_____ 17. During an argument I am sometimes afraid that I will get so upset that I will shake all over.

_____ 18. If a famed and respected lecturer makes a statement that I think is incorrect, I will have the audience hear my point of view.

_____ 19. I avoid arguing over prices with clerks and salespeople.

_____ 20. When I have done something important or worthwhile, I manage to let others know about it.

_____ 21. I am open and frank about my feelings.

_____ 22. If someone has been spreading false stories about me, I visit with him or her as soon as possible.

_____ 23. I often have a hard time saying no.

_____ 24. I tend to bottle up my emotions rather than make a scene.

_____ 25. I complain about poor service in a restaurant and elsewhere.

_____ 26. When I am given a compliment, I sometimes just don't know what to say.

Assessing Assertive Behavior *(cont'd)*

_____ 27. If a couple near me in a theater or at a lecture are conversing rather loudly, I ask them to be quiet or to take their conversation elsewhere.

_____ 28. Anyone attempting to push ahead of me in a line is in for a good battle.

_____ 29. I am quick to express an opinion.

_____ 30. There are times when I just can't say anything.

_____

Note: Adapted from "A 30 item schedule for assessing assertive behavior" by S. A. Rathus, 1973, *Behavior Therapy*, 4, 398–406. Copyright 1973 with permission from Elsevier.

FEEDBACK ON WORKSHEET 4.3

To score this scale, first change (reverse) the signs (+ or −) for your scores on items 1, 2, 4, 5, 9, 11, 12, 13, 14, 15, 16, 17, 19, 23, 24, 26, and 30. Now total the plus (+) items, total the minus (−) items, and subtract the minus total from the plus total to obtain your score. This score can range from −90 through 0 to +90.

The higher the score (closer to +90), the more assertively you usually behave. The lower the score (closer to −90), your typical behavior is more nonassertive. This particular scale does not measure aggressiveness.

No large-scale normative studies have been done on college students, and as such, limited normative data are available. However, one study with undergraduate students (Hull & Hull, 1978) found that the mean total score on this scale was 9.00 (standard deviation = 23.86) for males and 2.75 (standard deviation = 22.07) for females. Look at your score and see if you are above or below the mean.

What are some techniques the assertive person can practice to possibly prevent aggression or becoming too assertive? What are some practices for the nonassertive student? Stress levels are related to assertiveness or nonassertiveness—how will either behavior impact the student's life?

Five Steps to Becoming More Assertive

The following is a step-by-step process to become more assertive. Find a quiet place to work on this worksheet.

STEP 1. IDENTIFICATION OF AN ENVIRONMENTAL SITUATION

Identify an environmental situation for which you want feedback. It may be your work situation, or it may be your personal life or something else.

_____

_____

STEP 2. BEHAVIOR STYLE CLASSIFICATION

Identify and circle one of the following as your style of interpersonal behavior:

▨ *Passive.* Avoids problems, allows manipulation by others, gives up one's rights, and lacks self-confidence. This type of behavior is stress producing.

▨ *Assertive.* Faces problems, gains respect from others by letting them know one's opinions, claims rights, and has self-confidence. This type of behavior is least stress producing.

▨ *Aggressive.* Attacks the other person, takes advantage of people, disregards the rights of others, and is often hostile. This type of behavior is most stress producing.

Reasons:

_____

_____

_____

_____

STEP 3. PERSON IDENTIFICATION

All situations involve interacting with others. Identify the persons with whom you would like to be more assertive.

_____

_____

_____

_____

STEP 4. SCRIPT WRITING

Write a script for changing your actions and reactions in order to become more assertive with these people.

    a Identify your rights and feelings—define your goal.

_____

_____

Five Steps to Becoming More Assertive *(cont'd)*

_____

_____

_____

b Describe your feelings by using "I" statements. For example, "I like to … ," "I will … "

_____

_____

_____

_____

STEP 5. DISCUSSION SESSION

Have a discussion with the person with whom you would like to be more assertive, using the following checklist:

▨ Arrange a time and place for discussion.

▨ Concisely *define* the problem.

▨ *Describe* your feelings in "I" messages.

▨ Make your *request* in a brief sentence or two.

▨ *Reinforce* the other person's thinking by stating positive consequences of cooperation and, if necessary, negative consequences for failure to cooperate.

▨ Use assertive *body language* such as direct eye contact, erect body posture, and clarity of speech.

▨ Avoid manipulation.

▨ Be willing to compromise if it is essential.

references and further readings

Allessandra, T., O'Connor, M. J., & Allessandra, J. (1990). *People smart: Powerful techniques for turning every encounter into a mutual win.* La Jolla, CA: Keynote.

Berlo, D. K. (1960). *The process of communication.* New York: Holt, Rinehart and Winston.

Bower, S. A., & Bower, G. H. (1976). *Asserting yourself.* Reading, MA: Addison-Wesley.

Burke, C. R., Hall, D. R., & Hawley, D. (1986). *Living with stress.* Clackamas, OR: Wellsource.

Carlson Learning Company. (1994). *The Personal Profile System.* Minneapolis: Carlson Learning Company.

Covey, S. R. (1990). *The 7 habits of highly effective people.* Riverside, NJ: Simon & Schuster.

Davis, M., Eshelman, E. R., & McKay, M. (1982). *The relaxation and stress reduction workbook* (2nd ed.). Oakland, CA: New Harbinger.

Green, L. W., & Kreuter, M. W. (2005). *Health promotion planning: An educational and environmental approach* (4th ed.). Boston: McGraw-Hill.

Greenberg, J. S. (2010). *Comprehensive stress management* (12th ed.). Boston: Brown/McGraw-Hill.

Hull, D. B., & Hull, J. H. (1978). Rathus assertiveness schedule: Normative and factor analysis data. *Behavior Therapy, 9,* 673.

Kaufman, D., & O'Connor, M. J. (1992). *Basic questions and answer guide for needs motivated behavior.* Minneapolis: Carlson Marketing Group.

Kovacek, P. R. (1981). *Stress stoppers: Managing stress effectively.* Detroit: Henry Ford Hospital.

Lazarus, A. A. (1966). Behaviour rehearsal vs. nondirective therapy vs. advice in effecting behaviour change. *Behaviour Research and Therapy, 4,* 209–212.

Marston, W. M. (1979). *Emotions of normal people.* Minneapolis: Personal Press.

Mucchielli, R. (1970). *Introduction to structural psychology.* New York: Funk & Wagnalls.

Myers, P., & Nance, D. (1991). *The upset book* (2nd ed.). Wichita, KS: Mac Press.

O'Connor, M. J., & Merwin, S. J. (1992). *The mysteries of motivation: Why people do the things they do.* Minneapolis: Carlson Learning Company.

Performax Systems International. (1986). *The personal profile system manual and behavioral patterns master guide.* Minneapolis: Carlson Learning Company.

Rathus, S. A. (1973). A 30 item schedule for assessing assertive behavior. *Behavior Therapy, 4,* 398–406.

Robbins, S. P. & Judge, T. A. (2012). *Organizational behavior.* (15th ed.). Paramus, NJ: Prentice Hall.

Rokeach, M. (1970). *Beliefs, attitudes and values.* San Francisco: Jossey Bass.

Scott, E. (2011). Communicate: Improve your relationships with effective communication skills. Retrieved from http://stress.about.com/od/relationships/ht/healthycomm.htm

Selye, H. (1956). *The stress of life.* New York: McGraw-Hill.

Simonds, S. K. (1995). Communication theory and the search for effective feedback. *Journal of Human Hypertension, 9*(1), 5–10.

Smith, M. J. (1975). *When I say no, I feel guilty.* New York: Bantam Books.

Wolpe, J. (1958). *Psychotherapy by reciprocal inhibition.* Stanford, CA: Stanford University Press.

Yogananda, P. (1946). *Autobiography of a yogi.* Los Angeles: Self-Realization Fellowship.

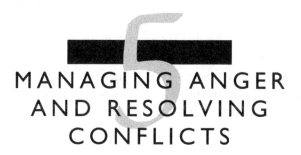

MANAGING ANGER AND RESOLVING CONFLICTS

Balancing your anger balances your life.

what is anger?

Anger is an emotion that, if not managed, neutralized, or controlled, can result in significant suffering for oneself, as well as for others. Frustration, a form of anger often results when we are not able to achieve a desired goal in a given time period. Feelings of anger are normal. However, uncontrolled anger results in release of various hormones and neurotransmitters. As a consequence, blood pressure rises, cardiac muscles contract, and gastric secretions increase. Eventually, the by-products produced do not get used in the system and accumulate, causing harm to the body. This buildup can manifest itself in the form of various illnesses such as hypertension, peptic ulcer, and stroke. Psychologically, uncontrolled anger "poisons the mind" and makes us perform actions that we may regret later. At the societal level, anger is at the root of many wars, terrorist activities, riots, looting, arson, domestic abuse, road rage, workplace violence, divorce, and so on. Therefore, anger that originates within the mind gradually engulfs the body, the family, and eventually has devastating effects on society. However, some anger within limits and with full awareness is beneficial because it protects the human organism. The key, however, is to have balance with anger. In this chapter, we will discuss how to attain this balance.

Many of us tend to "blow up" at the slightest provocation. Later, we regret our behavior when it is usually too late. According to Smith (1993), when considering anger, it is useful to begin by making some distinctions. Anger that results in aggression is destructive *behavior*. However, anger is essentially an internal *feeling*. While it is often appropriate to monitor and control aggressive behavior, feelings cannot always be controlled. It is necessary to realize that the feeling of anger can serve as a useful warning sign that we may be about to engage in aggressive or self-destructive behavior. Therefore, it is important to manage our anger and attain a "state of balance."

We have a number of diagnostic tests available for various medical disorders, but unfortunately no standard test is available for diagnosing anger. Moreover, a number of questions about anger continue to perplex and challenge us. For example, do we consider whether angry people are sick? Does getting angry make us feel better? If we let our anger out, what are the consequences? If we hold our anger in, what are the consequences?

managing the anger within

Most psychologists agree that if we become angry, we must feel that anger. There is no point in denying, hiding, repressing, or suppressing anger. This overt feeling is a natural process. We can appreciate that a newborn infant expresses these emotions of anger and rage by crying out at the time of birth. Throughout all ages or periods of development, many humans confront almost daily their own feelings of anger and those of other people with whom they come in contact. It is generally accepted today that we need anger to protect us from a hostile and aggressive world.

Unfortunately, we generally tend to do one of the following when experiencing anger within: (1) feel the anger but sit on it, deny it, and repress it; or (2) feel the anger and freely express it. Denial and repression of our anger does not get us anywhere, and "uncontrolled rage" leads to far more harm. Free expression of anger leads to hostility. Hostility is harmful for one's own health and that of others.

A well-known model to manage anger is based upon the concepts of rational emotive therapy (RET) developed by Albert Ellis (1975, 1977). He proposed the *hydraulic theory*, which states that anger and other emotions have a tendency to increase in intensity and expand under pressure like steam in a kettle. If we "squelch" our emotions and do not vent them, we run the risk of doing harm to ourselves. Real physical harm such as stomach ulcers, high blood pressure, or other ailments, including severe psychosomatic reactions, may result.

Conversely, if we let ourselves feel angry authentically (*free expression*) and let others know about our feelings, we may frequently encounter problems of quite another nature. People will react to our free expression of anger, in most instances, as an outwardly "aggressive or hostile" action and will probably close themselves off from us and defensively respond to us with further hostility. Venting anger freely is ineffective (Bushman, Baumeister, & Stack, 1999). Some therapists in the field have attempted to solve the problem with still another alternative, which they call *creative aggression* (or *constructive anger*). This response differs from the above free-expression method in that we express ourselves in a controlled and dignified manner and hope that others are willing to listen to our point of view.

We can appreciate that holding in and not expressing our anger is not a worthwhile idea. Free expression of anger also creates a whole complex of other counterproductive problems. Further, we have noted that creative aggression seems a more workable solution but that it still shares some of the same problems. According to Ellis (1977), another alternative, that of *unconditional forgiveness*, involves the "turning of the other cheek." This response seems somewhat inappropriate given the aggressive and sometimes hostile world in which we live.

According to Ellis (1977), anger begets anger. Therefore, the most practical solution in dealing with our anger is to become *annoyed* and *irritated*, so that we can become more effective at solving problems. To be annoyed is to be bothered. To be irritated is to become excited and provoked. Both these terms suggest a lowered level of emotional energy that has less impact on the body and mind. To become angry is to create more intense emotions that lead to greater consequences. We get angry and then try to fix the problem. Then, we get upset with our own anger. Subsequently, we develop a problem with the anger and its consequences. When we become angry, we usually either "let it out" or "hold it in." Another choice is to become annoyed and irritated; thus, we can solve problems. Ellis and Harper (1975) suggest that many people create irrational beliefs about what we should and should not do regarding anger. Research shows that when some people become angry, they need to reach closure immediately. For others, it is necessary to be alone, take time out, and work out the anger for themselves. Actually, in our culture we do not seem to have the best vocabulary to define those intense feelings we identify as anger. When people become angry, they often say, "You did that," rather than "I get annoyed when you do that."

Anger comes from a belief that the world should not be the way it is and should be the way I want it to be. This is actually an acknowledgment of the fact that all people have the freedom of will to choose to behave badly. If people do not have free will, then moral philosophy need not exist. When people behave badly, they have that right. No matter how many laws exist, no one can ever take away a person's free will. Ellis's school of thought suggests that we acknowledge and accept what others are by seeing these differences and becoming annoyed and irritated with these differences (Dryden & DiGiuseppe, 1990; Walen, DiGiuseppe, & Wessler, 1980). This annoyance and irritation on our part is often helpful in managing anger, for it helps us attain a balance (see Box 5.1, Tips on Managing Anger, Based on Eastern Philosophy, on page 102).

anger and stress: the connection

As shown in Chapter 1, the stress response has two components: *fight* and *flight*. The fight component of the stress response is a naturally occurring event, which is also responsible for angry behavior. Signs of anger and stress are interchangeable. Both anger and stress lead to anxiety, sleeplessness, uncontrolled thinking, brooding, restlessness, irritability, and so on. Along with these manifestations come headaches, muscle tension, peptic ulcers, and other stress-related problems. More dangerous are the reactions that we cannot feel (Eliot & Breo, 1989).

Another important dimension in the context of anger and stress is our personality. In people with Type A personalities, it appears that hostility and anger may be the key (Friedman & Rosenman, 1959, 1974; Lecic-Tosevski, Vukovic, & Stepanovic, 2011). We have already seen in Chapter 1 that people with Type A personalities experience greater stress. Coronary heart disease and essential hypertension are two serious diseases in particular that have been linked with anger. Some psychologists believe that hypertensives keep their blood pressure elevated by constantly suppressing their anger. According to Tavris (1982), "Release the anger, and blood pressure should fall." Another personality type that has been described in recent years is Type D (distressed) personality, which is characterized by a tendency toward negativity, low self esteem, and social inhibitions. Johan Denollet (2005) at Tilburg University, The Netherlands has developed a scale DS-14 to measure this Type D personality. These people experience a lot of stress, hostility, worry, tension and other negative emotions. People with Type D

BOX 5·1

Tips on Managing Anger, Based on Eastern Philosophy

Following are some helpful behavioral tips for managing anger within oneself. These are based on Eastern thought. We may want to reflect on some of these, and if we find any of these tips helpful, we should adopt them in our lives.

■ *Introspection* In any situation that makes us angry, there is always a component of our own responsibility. Therefore, we must always reflect on our contribution in triggering the anger. Any time we get angry, we should always try to find our mistake, no matter how little or trivial our contribution might have been. When we are angry or immediately after we have given way to anger, it is often not a good time for such "soul searching." However, once the mind has become a little calmer and, at the same time, not much time has elapsed since we got angry (not so much that we have forgotten all about it), we should perform this **introspection**. We should be critical of our own behavior and give the benefit of the doubt to the other party. Also, we should analyze the situation from the other person's point of view—we should try to step into the other person's shoes and look at the event triggering our anger from his or her perspective. Keeping these points in mind will help us decipher our own contribution toward anger.

■ *Apologizing and Determining to Rectify Our Contribution* Once we have identified our contribution in the situation that made us angry, if possible, we should make it a point to apologize to the other person without getting into any further argument. If

apologizing is not possible, we should make a conscious effort *not to repeat the same mistake* when we encounter a similar cue for action. We should repeat in our mind that we must not give way to anger the next time we are confronted with a similar situation. *Often in life, we repeat the same mistakes again and again.* Reflection on the root cause in any situation that triggers our anger oftentimes helps us decipher these repetitive patterns of mistakes. Developing a conscious awareness about these repetitive mistakes and fortifying the mind in dealing with them is often a helpful way to reduce the anger within ourselves in future encounters that have similar triggers.

■ *Understanding That Not Everything Can Be Changed, Fixed, or Altered* Often, our anger is directed toward another person or situation that cannot be changed, fixed, or altered. Understanding this reality of life and channeling our energies toward changing our own modifiable behaviors (which are frequently the only components that can be changed) are often helpful strategies that make us less angry.

■ *Letting Go* In present-day society, we have become overtly competitive in our disposition. We want to win at all cost, compete with others, covet the things that others have, and imagine that possessions will make us happier. Often these kinds of expectations are at the root of our anger. Remembering that life is not about competing with anyone but is about pursuing a journey of self-realization is indeed helpful in reducing anger in our lives.

---

personality are also prone to cardiovascular disease and a myriad of unhealthy behaviors (Mols & Denollet, 2010).

Anger also involves the feeling of pain and/or injury to oneself. If we personalize anger, we become fearful and anxious, feel cornered, become further angered, and lose control. This "loss of control" causes us to form judgments and make assumptions that further escalate our feeling of anger. To maintain balance and prevent anger from escalating, we need to preserve our self-worth, keep things in perspective, not unduly feed our fears, and *decide* to be in control of ourselves. *Thus, we reserve judgment and are able to maintain a problem-solving attitude.*

▨ An emotional response	Anger is an emotional reaction that normally happens in response to an unfulfilled desire, an unmet expectation, and an unimagined consequence.
▨ A warning signal	Anger helps us identify that something is wrong and is preventing us from achieving our goals.
▨ A way to new learning	Anger can facilitate our power of reflection and open a door to new learning, provided that we have an open mind and are willing to learn.
▨ A normal feeling	Anger is a normal response that all of us experience. It is not abnormal to be angry.
▨ Healthy within limits	Since anger is a feeling, if it is contained and not let out as a behavior, then it serves to release pent-up emotions. However, we need not deny, repress, or suppress anger for it to be healthy.
▨ A protective mechanism	Anger helps all living beings protect themselves from threatened surroundings and situations.
▨ Useful within limits	Anger helps us in setting interactive boundaries with people around us. It serves an important purpose in letting others appreciate what we like and what we dislike.

Anger is useful as a *signal* in which a "warning light" causes us to take action. As a solution, anger rarely helps, for it adds fuel to the fire, heats the problem, and may cause inappropriate behavior. See Thoughts for Reflection 5.1, What Anger Is, above, and Thoughts for Reflection 5.2, What Anger Is Not (page 104).

Expectations control our reactions to anger. That which we usually expect and which does not happen acts as a "triggering event" and causes a reaction to that which we seek a solution. The first time an expectation is not met, we have no idea how to approach the situation, so we think about what to do. If our solution seems to work, we try it out again in future situations. Once we are sure our solution works, we no longer wonder about whether it will work, and so we stop thinking about it and just do it. In this way, a habit is formed. If we have learned to react by getting angry, then we will react in that way irrespective of what the consequences will be. As time passes, reflection on the consequences decreases further and further. We also remind ourselves less and less about what it is that we are to do. Habituated response is an efficient way to operate, provided that the solution is really a good solution. In the case of anger, it is not a good solution. What really happens is that it causes a "fire," and we have to face the harmful consequences. This reaction needs to be changed. The following steps are to be considered in effecting this change:

1. Recognize and admit that your old solution (reaction) is not working.

2. Use the old reaction as a cue to start a search for a new solution.

3. Activate your thinking to identify the expectations upon which you are basing your reactions and begin to examine them critically.

Not a problem-solving tool	When we are angry, we should not attempt to solve problems, because anger does not help us in arriving at solutions. In fact, anger colors our perception, and we deviate from appropriate solutions.
Not an outlet for revenge	If anger is suppressed, it tends to make one vengeful, and revenge is not an appropriate response. It causes more harm than good.
Not blaming or projecting	We should not blame others for our anger, because anger is primarily an internal feeling that originates within our mind and has little to do with the outside world.
Not being violent	Anger is not an excuse for being violent. We should exercise adequate control of ourselves and our anger in not being violent, especially with innocent people, children, and so on.
Not a way of control	By being angry, we cannot control anyone else. We may, in the short run, create a sense of temporary fear that may look as if we have control, but in the long run it never works.
Not healthy if exceeds limits	Anger has been associated with a number of medical disorders, especially if it is uncontrolled.
Not useful if inappropriate	Anger is counterproductive. Anger loses its utility if we get angry too frequently or without proper reason.

4. Examine the validity of your expectations, reject those you find are not true or helpful, and replace them with **responses** that are.

5. With your expectations, the **response** will change.

6. Keep reinforcing new expectations and **responses** over and over again.

To manage the anger within, we need to identify situations in which we are likely to be angry. Then, we have to look for the *cues* for anger that trigger an event. *Unrealistic expectations are often at the root of most anger.* Understanding this root cause is helpful in reducing anger. Next we have to analyze the *costs* and *benefits* that come after our anger has subsided and the event is over. Managing anger mainly involves modifying these cues and consequences, and finding effective replacements (new responses) for the anger.

Therefore, the first step in managing anger is to find out where you are with anger in your personal life. **Worksheet 5.1** (page 116) has been designed to help you enhance this understanding of anger, and **Worksheet 5.2** (page 118) helps you manage anger.

dealing with an angry person

TRANSACTIONAL ANALYSIS

Eric Berne (1967) described a technique called **transactional analysis** (TA), a method for understanding interpersonal transactions. Transactions are defined as units of social intercourse.

An understanding of the basics of this method will enhance our skills to deal with anger within ourselves, as well as relate better with an angry person. According to transactional analysis, the various aspects of our personalities can be classified into three states:

1. *The Child Ego State* is the state in which we enter the world. Within the child ego state are three dimensions: (1) the *free child*, which is inquisitive, wants to have fun, be liked, and be admired; (2) the *rebellious child*, which has arisen because of certain experiences in childhood and rebels against domination; and (3) the *manipulative child*, which has developed as a result of learning some manipulative behavior in order to get needs fulfilled as children. An angry person is almost always in the child ego state (rebellious or manipulative). This ego state needs to be addressed first.

2. *The Parent Ego State* is the repository for events as we perceived them in the early years of our lives, up to 5 years of age. These recordings, or parent tapes, owe their origin to our parents and other significant people during our childhood who told us what to do and what not to do. These messages are resolved without editing and include all prohibitions, admonitions, and rules set by example or stated. The parent ego state has two parts: (1) the critical parent, which results in pronouncement of most imperatives like "you should," "you must," and "you ought to"; and (2) the nurturing or caring parent, which sympathizes, listens, encourages, and exhibits care and love.

3. *The Adult Ego State* is not synonymous with maturity. However, this state is the rational part of us and operates on data gathering and analysis. It is unemotional and helps us look at things through facts and objectivity.

The most intriguing aspect of this theory is that all of us possess these states within ourselves. With anger, we transcend into the child ego state. However, sometimes we may not appear childlike because we have camouflaged our feelings as either "critical parents," "caring parents," or "rational adults." If masquerading as a critical parent, we tend to use what we *should* have done or *ought* to be doing. In the mask of caring parent, we tend to be sarcastic. In the mask of a rational adult, we may try to give justification and rationalization that may actually be biased, and underneath might be a burning inferno. Besides other emotions such as worry and fear, bereavement may also appear like anger, but needs to be addressed in a different way.

With this understanding, it is clear that, when angry, a person is in a child ego state and this fact should be addressed first. It can be tackled by a caring parent response followed by a rational adult response. The problem occurs when we respond as a critical parent, evoke our child ego state, or move directly to the adult state, bypassing the caring parent. These responses do not extinguish anger but only make it flare up further. Evoking a caring parent response helps angry people be at ease and feel that their behavior has been addressed. When this is followed by a rational adult response, then understanding by an angry person of his or her "mistake(s)" is achieved. This approach helps disarm any angry person.

For example, a fellow student or fellow worker becomes angry with us about some event and stops speaking. If we do not speak to that person, it is likely to add to the existing anger. However, if we approach that person with a caring attitude and inquire about the reason for his anger, it is likely that he will tell us about the precipitating event from his perspective. Having reestablished rapport and gained understanding about the problem from the other person's perspective, we can

■ The troubles of our proud and angry dust are from eternity, and shall not fail. Bear them we can, and if we can we must. Shoulder the sky, my lad, and drink your ale.

—*A. E. Housman*

■ Anger is never without an argument, but seldom with a good one.

—*George Savile,
Marquis of Halifax*

■ Anger is one of the sinews of the soul. Anger makes a rich man hated and a poor man scorned.

—*Thomas Fuller*

■ Where it concerns himself,
Who's angry at a slander, makes it true.

—*Ben Jonson*

■ He that is slow to anger is better than the mighty; and he that ruleth his spirit than he that taketh a city.

—*Proverbs 16:32*

■ Anger makes dull men witty, but it keeps them poor.

—*Queen Elizabeth I*

■ Anger is a weed; hate is the tree.

—*St. Augustine*

■ In the depth of winter I finally learned that within me lay an invincible summer.

—*Albert Camus*

■ Anyone can become angry—that is easy. But to be angry with the right person, to the right degree, at the right time, for the right purpose, and in the right way—that is not easy.

—*Aristotle*

rationally analyze the situation and thus resolve the anger. Transactional analysis has been used in a variety of settings, such as to teach pharmacy students how to counsel patients (Lawrence, 2007) and to improve communication between faculty and students in nursing education (Keçeci & Taşocak, 2009). See Thoughts for Reflection 5.3, Points to Ponder, above.

THE TIME-OUT PROCEDURE

Often when we are angry, we do not think. To reactivate our thinking, we need to put aside everything in which we are engaged and find time to reflect and introspect. The time-out procedure detailed in this section (Coursol & Veenstra, 1986) provides us with the opportunity to reflect upon our actions, then accordingly change them. It consists of the following steps:

1. *Stop* We have to immediately put a stop to our conventional behavior. We can no longer react by getting angry in situations that angered us earlier. This determination to "stop" is the first step in the time-out procedure.

2. *Think* Having stopped our conventional reaction, we need to think about a new approach in dealing with situations that may provoke anger. Think about this new way by identifying and describing the new skills (responses) that will be required. Also think about the approaches and possible barriers in acquiring these new skills.

3. *Act* We need to overcome the cognitive barriers (i.e., faulty beliefs and expectations) that stand in the way of implementing the new way. Having overcome the barriers, act on the new way by practicing the new skills (responses).

The effectiveness of the time-out procedure is based upon the other person's view of the position we have taken. A person's perception is a factor in that once we attempt to practice the time-out procedure, it is up to the other person to respond to us. An angry person wants to get his or her point across to us so as to get relief from his or her sense of injustice. Relief also gives hope that the problem-solving process has started. What an angry person usually gets is a counterattack explaining why he or she was wrong. Because the "defense of self" is a priority, an angry person does not listen (Coursol & Veenstra, 1986). What an angry person does in response is defend the self and attack more intensely. The anger is increased because of the pain felt of not being understood. The angry person becomes apprehensive that the problem will continue unsolved. In the time-out procedure (Coursol & Veenstra, 1986), options that are helpful when listening to an angry person consist of the following:

❍ *Reflective or Empathic Listening* "What you are saying is . . ." In this approach, we are serving as a mirror, acknowledging what the other person is saying but not putting out our own view as a target. Our own viewpoint is preserved and set aside from consideration.

❍ *Possible Agreement or Fogging* "Let me think about that . . ." In this approach, we acknowledge that the other person might be on target, but we are not committing ourselves definitely. It is important to follow through on problem solving so the other person will not see it as a stall.

❍ *Actual Agreement or Admitting that We Are Wrong* "You are right, it was wrong for me to . . ." In this approach, we acknowledge that the other person is on target and admit that we are wrong and at fault. If we don't genuinely believe we are wrong, this will only "stuff" and not solve the problem.

❍ *Negative Inquiry or Inviting Further Criticism* "Are there other things I do that hurt you?" In this approach, we give an opportunity to have the other person aim at the target. This option must be done genuinely.

This valuable technique, which has been shown to manage anger effectively, is the time-out procedure shown in Figure 5.1.

THE "UPSET" PHILOSOPHY

According to Myers and Nance (1991), angry people are usually upset. Moreover, we also become upset when we have to deal with an angry person. We can cope with an angry person if we can identify and understand the specific incident that triggered the anger. We will also have success in preventing another person from becoming angry if we understand the kinds of situations that are likely to provoke anger.

Anger is the result of many factors, including a triggering or precipitating situation, our past experiences, individual responses to experiences, and idiosyncrasies. Understanding what creates anger in another person is often helpful both in planning preventive strategies and in deciding how to handle anger once it occurs. Therefore, we have to examine the situation of the other person. We have to step into the shoes of the other person and then look at the situation from his or her angle.

Myers and Nance (1991) have identified several triggering factors and events, as follows:

1. *Dependency* Usually a feeling of dependence on another person, object, or thing can lead to increased anger. Anger is especially accentuated when we

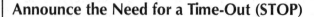

Announce the Need for a Time-Out (STOP)   **1**

- Indicate that you are feeling angry about the situation.
- Discuss the need for this time-out or time away from the situation.
- Leave the situation so as not to threaten others.

Take Time-Out to Assess the Situation (THINK)   **2**

- Work at calming down the bodily (psychophys-iological) reaction that is now apparent.
- Become more open to the views of others.

Coming Back after Taking Time-Out (ACT)   **3**

- Be willing to admit to self and especially others that you might have been a contributing factor in creating anger.
- Agree to work together to continue discussing problems.

Figure 5.1 The Time-Out Procedure

are intimately dependent and cannot find alternatives to our dependency. A person with such feelings can be helped by providing enough choices and helping that person become more independent.

2. *Authority* Authority normally comes by position, expertise, or wealth. Often-times authority makes a person inappropriately authoritarian. People who are authoritarian tend to utilize their authority in a manner that provokes anger. It is the way they say things that creates anger in others. It may not be what they say but how they say it that precipitates anger. Therefore, we need to be very careful in how we present a point of view and using our authority.

3. *Unclear Limits* Some of us want and seek direction in how we perform our tasks. These directions can come from our parents, our peers, our teachers, our employers, our colleagues, our spouses, and so on. When these directions are unclear, confusing, or dualistic, they lead to anger and frustration. Anger originating from this type of unclarity can be dealt with by setting specific directions and limits. If these directions come from within ourselves, then greater autonomy and control can be achieved in dealing with anger.

4. *Complexity* Many situations are apparently complicated, intricate, and com-plex. If we get stuck in the complexity, then we are prone to get angry. This type of anger can be tackled by simplifying the process by breaking it down into smaller parts or steps. Breaking down any complicated event into smaller parts or steps often simplifies the process. We need to constantly remember that life is essentially a simple process.

Once you have explored what anger is and its related causes, you can now think about how to defuse anger observed in others. Some suggested methods follow:

▓ *Listening Attentively.* Learn to listen first to another instead of over-reacting to a given situation. Avoid criticism and do not personalize what you hear. Also, avoid replying with an attack mode. It is important to seek out those areas of agreement for both parties.

▓ *Acknowledge Feelings.* Let the other person know you understand that they are expressing anger. Emphasize your understanding that they are angry and avoid telling them they should not have the feelings they have.

▓ *Agreeing.* Simply put, look for areas that each of you can agree upon. Avoid putting the other person down for expressing their discord and anger. Search out points that each of you have relevant to a common ground.

▓ *Problem Agreement.* Reach an understanding of what the actual problem is.

▓ *Identifying Solutions.* Once you have some agreement on what the problem is, brainstorm some solutions, then attempt to agree on one best solution.

▓ *Reaching Closure.* Genuinely thank the person for letting you know about their anger. Ask if there is anything else you could do and whether or not the other person is satisfied with the discussion. The key to reaching a valued solution is that both parties have an understanding of what the problem is.

5. *Prior Unresolved Conflict* Past events are an important source of our anger, especially events for which we have not reached closure or which have not been resolved amicably. These events and associated anger keep surfacing again and again. Until and unless these conflicts are completely resolved, sublimation of anger cannot result. We need to put our mind and effort toward resolving conflicts that we can resolve. We need to strengthen our mind to "forgive and forget" the conflicts over which we have no control.

6. *Communication Problems* We have seen in Chapter 4 that poor, ineffective, and marginal communication often leads to stress and anger. If we are not able to communicate effectively, this failure causes anger and frustration in us as well as others. This poor communication can result from a number of causes. Some of these causes may pertain to us, while some may pertain to others. Though we cannot do much about how others communicate, we can certainly improve upon our own communication, especially when this miscommunication is an intended one, for inexplicable reasons, on our part. As far as possible, we should try to identify these reasons, overcome them, and make our communication as clear and effective as possible.

7. *Conflict of Interest* People have different ideas and interests. Sometimes when a task needs to be achieved, these differences tend to be mutually conflicting. This **conflict** can be a source of anger and frustration. Therefore, all potential conflicts need to be resolved. Thoughts for Reflection 5.4, Resolving Conflicts by Managing Anger, and 5.5, Five Conflict-Handling Orientations (above and page 110, respectively) provides some suggestions for resolving conflicts.

**FIVE CONFLICT-
HANDLING
ORIENTATIONS**

Conflict-Handling Orientation	Appropriate Situations
1. Competition	When quick, decisive action is vital
	On the important issues where unpopular actions need implementing
	On issues vital to the organization's welfare and when you know you're right
	Against people who take advantage of noncompetitive behavior
2. Collaboration	To find an integrative solution when both sets of concerns are too important to be compromised
	When your objective is to learn
	To merge insights from people with different perspectives
	To gain commitment by incorporating concerns into a consensus
	To work through feelings that have interfered with a relationship
3. Avoidance	When an issue is trivial, or more important issues are pressing
	When you perceive no chance of satisfying your concerns
	When potential disruption outweighs the benefits of resolution
	To let people cool down and regain perspective
	When gathering information supersedes immediate decision
	When others can resolve the conflict more effectively
	When issues seem tangential or symptomatic of other issues
4. Accommodation	When you find you are wrong, to allow a better position to be heard, to learn, and to show your reasonableness
	When issues are more important to others than yourself, to satisfy others and maintain cooperation
	To build social credits for later issues
	To minimize loss when you are outmatched and losing
	When harmony and stability are especially important
	To allow subordinates to develop by learning from mistakes
5. Compromise	When goals are beneficial but not worth the effort or potential disruption of more assertive modes
	When opponents with equal power are committed to mutually exclusive goals
	To achieve temporary settlements to complex issues
	To arrive at expedient solutions under time pressure
	As a backup when collaboration or competition is unsuccessful

Note: From "Toward Multidimensional Values in Teaching: The Example of Conflict Behaviors" By K. W. Thomas, July 1977, *Academy of Management Review*, P. 487. Copyright 1977 by Academy of Management Review. Reprinted by Permission.

1. Do not take anger personally. Maintain a sense of self-worth. Ask yourself:
   - "Are they having a rough day?"
   - "Is this really directed at me?"
   - "Are they just criticizing my behavior, not my being?"

2. Keep anger in perspective. Do not feed your fears. Tell yourself:
   - "Relax, you can make it through this."
   - "It is not going to be the end of the world."
   - "It is not that bad."

3. Decide to be in control of yourself. Repeat to yourself:
   - "I shall not let the anger control me."
   - "I can and will control the anger."

4. Do not be judgmental. Ask yourself:
   - "Do I need to attribute reasons?"
   - "Am I expecting too much in this situation?"
   - "Can anyone always win?"

5. Maintain a problem-solving attitude. Ask yourself:
   - "Do I have an open mind?"
   - "What are the alternatives?"

ACTIVE LISTENING

An important factor in managing anger is the ability to "listen actively." Active listening is an intervention that addresses our interaction with others (Steinmetz, Blankenship, Brown, Hall, & Miller, 1980). This is an effective yet simple tool for managing anger and thereby reducing stress. Its application is very versatile.

First, active listening is a *diagnostic tool*. It helps one identify and pinpoint the cause or reason for the other person's anger. Second, active listening is a *disarming device* that helps the angry person to appropriately "let out" his or her feelings. Third, active listening provides an opportunity to seek *clarification*, which is an essential component for resolving anger. Fourth, active listening aids to *rationalize*, develop *clear thinking*, and *communicate effectively* in order to mutually resolve anger. Finally, active listening helps the angry person preserve his or her *dignity* and not express anger in an undignified manner.

Worksheet 5.3 (page 120) has been designed to help you deal more effectively with an angry person through active listening. Since this work sheet involves role playing, it cannot be completed alone and requires the cooperation of a partner.

For further discussion of the issues involved in managing anger and resolving conflict, see Thoughts for Reflection 5.6, Calming Reminders (above), Box 5.2, The Growing Menace of Violence (page 112), and Thoughts for Reflection 5.7, The Value of "I" Messages (page 113).

BOX 5·2

The Growing Menace of Violence

Violence is becoming more and more pervasive in our society, whether it is at a personal, family, school, national, or global level. Not a single day goes by when we do not encounter news items such as " boy brings a gun to school and threatens classmates" or "spouse is beaten by enraged partner" or "teenage driver under road rage critically injures a pedestrian" or a "suicide bomber kills so many people in some part of the world" or "a country launches an attack on another nation." We, as consumers of these news items, are fascinated by violence-related news stories, perhaps because they seem to justify our own indiscretions or fantasies. In any event, violence in our society has reached levels that are a threat to public health. We have to remember that the root cause of all violence is anger.

Anger at a personal level escalates into violent situations for self and others and contributes to disharmony at societal levels. At the *first* level, family violence and abuse is very common in our society. Family violence includes abuse and neglect of children, spousal abuse, sibling rivalries, abuse of elderly, and violence between separated or divorced partners (Barzelatto, 1998; Walden, 2002). Violence in family situations can manifest as physical abuse, sexual abuse, emotional abuse, verbal abuse, or economical abuse. Improved communication skills, problem-solving skills, and conflict resolution skills, discussed in this and the previous chapter, are indispensable in dealing with violence of this nature.

At the *second* level, violence occurs at community-group levels such as in schools, in neighborhood gangs, and at worksites. Manifestations of this level of violence cover a wide range of consequences, from verbal threats to homicides. Availability and proliferation of firearms and action movies have also aided to increase this level of violence. Recent years have seen two saddening trends with this kind of violence. The first trend is the involvement of younger and younger children. The second is the irreversible deadly consequences as a result of these violent acts, primarily due to sophistication of firearms. Political will to develop robust policies that restrict such violence and effective enforcement of these policies is needed, in addition to the various individual-level measures discussed previously to prevent and curb individual-level anger and violence (Sanderford-O'Connor, 2002).

The *third* and *final* level of violence is at national and international levels in which nations and ideologies clash, mostly for power and dominance. Growing disparities between "haves" and "have-nots" and the inability to find solutions through negotiations, compromises, adjustments, and altering a desired course of action are all contributory factors to violence between nations. Although nothing more than wishful thinking can be done at the personal level to solve this problem, nonetheless, if a critical mass of "wishful thinkers"—who believed in and promoted universal harmony—was created, a change in the global world order might not be difficult to achieve.

If you start a statement with an "I," it implies you are owning responsibility. If you start a statement with "you," that implies that you are shifting responsibility to the other person. Every "you" message can be turned into an "I" message; then it becomes a nonblaming statement about one's own self. Of course, you cannot talk in calm "I" messages all the time. There is no distinct advantage in using "I" messages for all situations. If your goal is to let the other person know that you are angry, you can do it in your own personal style, and your style may do the job. If, however, your goal is to break a pattern in a significant relationship and/or to develop a stronger

sense of self that you can bring to all your relationships, it is essential that you learn to translate your anger into clear, nonblaming statements about yourself—that is, "I" statements (Lerner, 1985).

Here are some examples of how you can turn some common "you" statements into "I" statements. We commonly say "You argue with me." This can be changed to "When I am talking with you, we argue." Another "you" statement is "You yell at me." This can be modified as "When I am talking with you, we get loud." Yet another one is "You annoy me." This can be changed to "When I am talking to you, I get annoyed."

CHAPTER REVIEW

summary points

- ○ Unmanaged anger is harmful to self and others.

- ○ Anger is an internal *feeling* that, if not managed, results in aggression, which is a destructive *behavior*.

- ○ Denying, repressing, or even freely expressing anger is often harmful.

- ○ In order to manage anger within ourselves, through rational emotive therapy as described by Albert Ellis, we need to become *annoyed* and *irritated*. This annoyance and irritation help us to attain balance with anger.

- ○ Unfulfilled and unrealistic expectations are at the root of anger. An understanding of these often leads to decreased anger.

- ○ Instead of reacting to anger from habit, we can choose to respond appropriately to valid expectations.

- ○ Transactional analysis, first described by Eric Berne, is a useful technique in dealing with an angry person.

- ○ According to transactional analysis, our personalities have three ego states: child (free, rebellious, manipulative), parent (critical, caring), and adult (rational).

- ○ A caring parent response followed by a rational adult response is often helpful in extinguishing the anger of an angry person.

- ○ The time-out procedure, or giving oneself adequate time to reflect and introspect on dealing with an angry person, is often a helpful approach.

o The "upset" philosophy, described by Myers and Nance, recognizes several triggering factors for anger: dependency, authority, unclear limits, complexity, prior unresolved conflict, communication problems, and conflict of interest.

o Five conflict-handling orientations are competition, collaboration, avoidance, accommodation, and compromise.

o Active listening is an effective tool to disarm any angry person. It involves direct questioning, rationalizing, clarifying, and supporting.

important terms defined

anger: A normal emotion one encounters when presented with an obstacle or difficulty in accomplishing a desired goal in a desired way in a desired time frame.

conflict: A situation involving anger between two or more people.

introspection: A self-analysis process exploring the reasons and motivations behind one's own behaviors.

transactional analysis: An interpersonal analysis technique based on assumption of three ego states—child, parent, and adult—within each individual.

websites to explore

AMERICAN PSYCHOLOGICAL ASSOCIATION

www.apa.org/topics/anger/control.aspx

This website from the American Psychological Association provides specific information about controlling anger.

▦ Explore this website and make a personal five-point plan to reduce anger in your life.

ANGER ALTERNATIVES

www.anger.org/

This website provides information about a group, Anger Alternatives, that supports and trains people to stop reactionary and violent behaviors.

▦ Explore this website and summarize the chief activities of this group.

ANGER MANAGEMENT

www.angriesout.com/

This website from a group called Talk, Trust, and Feel Therapeutics introduces the work of Lynne Namke. It provides ideas for alternatives to conflict and violence when one is upset.

▦ Explore the links on this website. What alternatives to anger were you able to find?

ANGER MANAGEMENT HOME STUDY COURSE

www.angermgmt.com/

This website provides information about a continuing education course in anger management for professionals seeking additional insights and techniques for dealing with the anger of their clients.

▦ Read about the home study course and see if you are interested in doing it.

CONFLICT RESOLUTION

http://helpguide.org/mental/eq8_conflict_resolution.htm

This website provides information about conflict resolution techniques. It describes understanding conflict in relationships, unhealthy and healthy responses to conflict, successful methods for resolving conflicts, and related articles and resources.

■ Read the information provided on this website, explore a few additional resources listed, and make a list of ten points to resolve conflicts. Apply those points to a conflict situation that you might be having.

WORKSHEET 5.1

This worksheet is available online at www.pearsonhighered.com/romas.

Self-Assessment of Anger

Respond to the following questions honestly. Your reactions will serve as a means of feedback for your own improvement in managing anger.

1. Is anger a problem for me? _____ Yes _____ No _____ Not sure

2. How do I know when I am angry?

_____

_____

_____

_____

_____

_____

3. How do I feel inside when I am angry?

_____

_____

_____

_____

_____

_____

4. What do I do about my anger?

_____

_____

_____

_____

_____

_____

Self-Assessment of Anger *(cont'd)*

5. Describe the last time you got angry. At what or with whom were you angry? How did this affect you?

_____

_____

_____

_____

_____

6. Analyze your reasons for becoming angry.

_____

_____

_____

_____

_____

7. Indicate any problems created by your anger.

_____

_____

_____

_____

_____

_____

FEEDBACK ON WORKSHEET 5.1

Worksheet 5.1 helps you to acquire a greater insight into the situations and persons with whom you become angry. If you can identify the situations that cause your anger and the various negative consequences that you have to face as a result of your anger, you can become more motivated to change your behavior. This enhanced awareness is the basis of, and the first step toward changing, your reaction to anger.

WORKSHEET 5.2

This worksheet is available online at www.pearsonhighered.com/romas.

Managing Your Anger

This worksheet is designed to help you deal with your anger in a more productive way. Seek out a quiet place to reflect upon and respond to the following statements.

1. Identify a situation in which you have expressed anger inappropriately. Analyze your goals and/or desired expectations. Then break the situation down into steps. Examine at which step the anger became apparent.

Situation:

_____

_____

_____

_____

Goals/desired expectations:

_____

_____

Steps in the event:

_____

_____

_____

_____

_____

2. Describe the benefits this anger had.

_____

_____

_____

_____

3. Did the anger cost you anything or cause any harm?

_____

_____

_____

_____

Managing Your Anger *(cont'd)*

4. Did the costs outweigh the benefits? _____ Yes _____ No

5. What alternative step(s) could you have taken instead of the one in which you got angry and still met your goal/desired expectations?

_____

_____

_____

_____

_____

6. What were the barriers that prevented you from adopting this alternative step?

_____

_____

_____

_____

_____

7. How can you overcome these barriers in the future?

_____

_____

_____

_____

_____

Learning Active Listening

To practice active listening, you will require the cooperation of a partner. This activity involves role playing and sharpening your skills to listen actively. Ask your partner to imagine a situation in which he or she was or will be angry with you. Let him or her imagine that situation mentally. You, as well as your partner, will have to work at this role play. Following are some of the guidelines for you to work on.

Self	Partner
Direct questioning: Start probing the reasons for your partner's anger in a calm and controlled manner.	Since you are angry, you may choose to respond or not respond.
Rationalizing: Try to understand your partner's feelings. Also try to understand the reasons and explanations for this behavior in your own mind.	Act out the way you actually feel.
Clarifying: You may want to seek clarification on your partner's feelings and responses.	Behave the way you feel.
Supporting: As much as possible, try to support your partner's viewpoint. This may be difficult.	You may choose whether or not to yield to the responses.

FEEDBACK ON WORKSHEET 5.3

Both you and your partner need to focus on the way you are feeling now. Has the anger been resolved? If so, discuss the reasons. If not, discuss why not. You may want to write some of your learnings from this experience in the space below.

_____

_____

_____

_____

_____

_____

You may want to reinforce these learnings from time to time so that they become a part of your behavior, and then you can deal with an angry person more effectively. Your partner may want to change roles with you and improve his or her ability to deal with angry people.

references and further readings

Barzelatto, J. (1998). Understanding sexual and reproductive violence: An overview. *International Journal of Gynaecology and Obstetrics, 63* (Suppl. 1), 13–18.

Berne, E. (1967). *Transactional analysis.* New York: Harper College.

Bushman, B. J., Baumeister, R. F., & Stack, A. D. (1999). Catharsis, aggression, and persuasive influence: Self-fulfilling or self-defeating prophecies? *Journal of Personality and Social Psychology, 76*(3), 367–376.

Coursol, D., & Veenstra, G. (1986). *Anger control.* Unpublished manuscript, University of Kansas School of Medicine, Wichita.

Davis, M., Eshelman, E. R., & McKay, M. (2008). *The relaxation and stress reduction workbook* (6th ed.). Oakland, CA: New Harbinger.

Denollet, J. (2005). DS14: Standard assessment of negative affectivity, social inhibition, and Type D personality. *Psychosomatic Medicine, 67*(1), 89–97.

Dryden, W., & DiGiuseppe, R. (1990). *A primer on rational-emotive therapy.* Champaign, IL: Research Press.

Eliot, R. S., & Breo, D. L. (1989). *Is it worth dying for? How to make stress work for you—not against you.* New York: Bantam.

Ellis, A. (1975). *How to live with a neurotic.* North Hollywood, CA: Wilshire.

Ellis, A. (1977). *Anger: How to live with and without it.* Secaucus, NJ: Citadel Press.

Ellis, A., & Harper, R. A. (1975). *A new guide to rational living.* North Hollywood, CA: Wilshire.

Friedman, M., & Rosenman, R. H. (1959). Association of specific overt behavior pattern with blood and cardiovascular findings: Blood clotting time, incidence of arcus senilis, and clinical coronary artery disease. *Journal of the American Medical Association, 169,* 1286–1296.

Friedman, M., & Rosenman, R. H. (1974). *Type A behavior and your heart.* New York: Fawcett Crest.

Greenberg, J. S. (2008). *Comprehensive stress management* (10th ed.). Boston: McGraw-Hill.

Keçeci, A., & Taşocak, G. (2009). Nurse faculty members' ego states: transactional analysis approach. *Nurse Education Today, 29*(7), 746–752.

Lawrence, L. (2007). Applying transactional analysis and personality assessment to improve patient counseling and communication skills. *American Journal of Pharmaceutical Education, 71*(4), 81.

Lecic-Tosevski, D., Vukovic, O., & Stepanovic, J. (2011). Stress and personality. *Psychiatrike, 22*(4), 290–297.

Lerner, H. G. (1985). *The dance of anger.* New York: Harper & Row.

Mols, F., & Denollet, J. (2010). Type D personality in the general population: A systematic review of health status, mechanisms of disease, and work-related problems. *Health and Quality of Life Outcomes, 8,* 9.

Myers, P., & Nance, D. (1991). *The upset book* (2nd ed.). Wichita, KS: Mac Press.

Sanderford-O'Connor, V. (2002). Violence prevention techniques for over-stressed workplaces. *Occupational Health and Safety, 71,* 102–105.

Smith, J. C. (1993). *Creative stress management: The 1–2–3 cope system.* Englewood Cliffs, NJ: Prentice Hall.

Steinmetz, J., Blankenship, J., Brown, L., Hall, D., & Miller, G. (1980). *Managing stress before it manages you.* Palo Alto, CA: Bull.

Tavris, C. (1982). *Anger: The misunderstood emotion.* New York: Simon & Schuster.

Thomas, K. W. (1977, July). Toward multidimensional values in teaching: The example of conflict behaviors. *Academy of Management Review,* 487.

Walden, R. J. (2002). Domestic violence. *Journal of the Royal Society of Medicine, 95,* 427.

Walen, S. R., DiGiuseppe, R., & Wessler, R. L. (1980). *A practitioner's guide to rational-emotive therapy.* New York: Oxford University Press.

COPING WITH ANXIETY

STRESS
MANAGEMENT
PRINCIPLE

" Wipe out anxiety before it wipes you out. "

what is anxiety?

Anxiety is an inevitable part of life. Inherent in anxiety are two components—inefficiency and fear. *Inefficiency* is the loss of one's mental alertness and inability to gear the mind toward problem solving. To *fear* is to imagine that one's own actions always have bad or painful consequences or to imagine only possible adverse events (Maharishi, 1989). Greenberg (2010) has described anxiety, operationally, as an unrealistic fear resulting in physiological arousal and accompanied by the behavioral signs of escape or avoidance. When this feeling of anxiety becomes uncontrolled or excessive, then it knocks one down. Various mental disorders are associated with excessive anxiety. *Generalized anxiety disorder* is characterized by unrealistic or excessive anxiety and worry about life situations (Culpepper, 2002; Piero, 2010). Some of the symptoms of this disorder are (*Diagnostic and Statistical Manual of Mental Disorders—DSM IV–TR*, 2000):

1. Trembling, twitching, feeling shaky

2. Muscle tension, aches, soreness

3. Restlessness

4. Easy fatigability

5. Shortness of breath

6. Palpitations, feeling of heart beating faster

7. Sweating

8. Dryness of mouth

9. Dizziness, light-headedness

10. Nausea

11. Flushes

12. Frequent urination

13. Trouble in swallowing, "lump in throat"

14. Feeling "keyed up" or "on edge"

15. Difficulty concentrating

16. Irritability

17. Trouble falling or staying asleep

In some rural areas and subpopulations of the United States, patients use unique expressions to describe anxiety, such as "I got the churnings," "I'm uptight," or "I am always freaking out" (Shader & Greenblatt, 1993).

Another type of anxiety disorder is *panic disorder*. The key symptoms associated with panic attacks are (DSM IV–TR, 2000):

1. Shortness of breath, smothering sensation

2. Dizziness, unsteady feelings, or faintness

3. Palpitations

4. Trembling, shaking

5. Sweating

6. Choking

7. Nausea, abdominal distress

8. Depersonalization, derealization

9. Numbness, tingling sensations

10. Flushes

11. Chest pain

12. Fear of dying

13. Fear of going crazy or doing something uncontrolled

Panic disorders may occur alone or in conjunction with a secondary syndrome termed *agoraphobia*, a fear of being in places or situations from which escape might be difficult, embarrassing, or in which help might not be available in the event of a panic attack. Affected persons usually restrict their travel or need a companion when they are away from home or familiar places. The severity of avoidance behavior can range from mild, in which there is distress, to severe, in which the person is completely homebound.

Some other anxiety disorders include (DSM IV–TR, 2000):

1. *Specific phobias*, which consist of excessive or unreasonable fear of a specific object or situation (for example, elevators, flying, heights, or some type of animal).

2. *Social phobias*, which include a marked and persistent fear of social or performance situations (for example, public speaking, entering a room full of strangers, or using a public restroom).

3. *Obsessive compulsive disorders (OCD)*, which consist of obsessions and compulsions. *Obsessions* are recurrent and persistent thoughts, impulses, or images that are intrusive and inappropriate and cause anxiety. *Compulsions* are urgent repetitive behaviors such as hand washing, counting, or repeatedly checking to make sure that some dreaded event will not occur (for example, checking that all doors are locked and then checking again and again).

4. *Posttraumatic stress disorder (PTSD)*, in which a person has been exposed to an event that involved actual or threatened death or serious injury, and the person reacted with intense fear, helplessness, or horror. In this disorder, the person persistently re-experiences the event through recollections, dreams, or a sudden feeling as if it were recurring. See Box 6.1, Stress and the Events of 9/11 (page 126).

Population-based surveys about emotional disorders in the United States have revealed a one-year period of prevalent anxiety among adults between 5 and 15 percent and panic disorders between 1 and 2 percent (Chou et al, 2011; Kessler & Wittchow, 2002; Regier et al., 1988).

These are, however, representations of pathological conditions that require treatment with benzodiazepines and other drugs. In this chapter, we learn about mechanisms that can prevent these conditions from occurring. Prevention requires systematic and regular practice in order to cope with worrying and anxiety so that these feelings do not get out of proportion and result in disorders. By learning these practical techniques, one can reduce worrying and anxiety and maintain long-lasting health and happiness in life.

Before you proceed to learn these techniques, take the Taylor Manifest Anxiety Scale in **Worksheet 6.1** (page 136), which measures the degree to which you manifest anxiety.

The Taylor Manifest Anxiety Scale measures what is known as **trait anxiety**. If your score is over 35 in the Taylor scale, it indicates that your anxiety is evidencing itself in physical and/or psychological symptoms and warrants serious attention (Allen & Hyde, 1980). Therefore, it is necessary for you to master the techniques presented in this chapter. The other type of anxiety is **state anxiety**, which is temporary in nature and is usually associated with a stimulus. State anxiety is situation specific. The techniques presented in this chapter, when practiced over a long time, will also help in coping with state anxiety See Thoughts for Reflection 6.1, When You Worry, Think! (page 127).

depression

Besides anxiety, sometimes a person may also manifest depression. The classical signs and symptoms of depression include the presence of five or more of the following (DSM IV–TR, 2000):

1. Depressed mood most of the day, nearly every day

2. Diminished interest or pleasure in most activities

3. Significant changes in body weight or appetite (increased or decreased)

Stress and the Events of 9/11

On September 11, 2001, terrorists on a suicide mission hijacked four American passenger jets. They flew two of them into the World Trade Center, causing the twin towers in New York City to crumple to earth. Another plane smashed into the Pentagon outside Washington, DC. The fourth plane crashed in Shanksville, Pennsylvania, instead of hitting its intended target—the White House or Capitol. The aftershocks of these acts of terrorism caused unparalleled stress among Americans and other people around the world.

The attacks made all of us ponder our own vulnerabilities. The magnitude of the destruction and the level of organization that produced it made ordinary Americans look at security from a totally new perspective. Previously unfamiliar feelings of suspicion and fear gripped us as we wondered whether terrorists were living in our midst and might strike again. Reported cases of anxiety-related disorders—particularly post-traumatic stress disorder (PTSD)—rose to high levels. All these were signs of societal stress.

Are such stress and anxiety preventable? Perhaps. The greatest stress arises out of individuals' imagining their own vulnerability to the stressors. Even though the events of 9/11 were once-in-a-lifetime events, we tend to overestimate the likelihood that they will happen again. Why do we do this? Why do our fears become so powerful? We lose perspective. We forget an important stress management principle: It is not the stressor but the perception of the stress that is important.

Terrorist acts are not uncommon around the world. Hardly any day passes without a terrorist somewhere bringing destruction to property and human life. Yet the overwhelming majority of people never experience terrorism. At the beginning of this century, the population of the world reached 6 billion, and the number keeps growing. Even the U.S. population of about 314 million is quite large. Events as horrific as the attacks of 9/11 are rare phenomena that directly affect very few individuals. We all know that thousands of flights take place safely every day, and we are not likely to find ourselves the victims of terrorist activity in the air or on the ground.

We need to stay aware of the relationship between media coverage of momentous events and our levels of stress. Repeated viewing of television coverage fuels our anxiety and leads us to erroneously dread the recurrence of highly unlikely events. Why do we choose to watch replays of tragic events? We know the media are not reluctant to frighten us. Perhaps we subconsciously like to harbor fear.

In the aftermath of 9/11, we need to remember the importance of realistically appraising life-event stressors so that we can manage the stress in our lives.

---

4. Insomnia or hypersomnia nearly every day

5. Psychomotor agitation (increased activity) or retardation (decreased activity)

6. Fatigue or loss of energy

7. Feelings of worthlessness or excessive guilt

8. Diminished ability to think or concentrate

9. Recurrent thoughts of death or suicide, attempt or plan to commit suicide

A *depressive illness* is a whole-body illness, involving your body, mood, thoughts, and behavior. It affects the way you eat and sleep, the way you feel about yourself, and the way you think about things. A depressive illness is *not* a passing blue mood. It is *not* a sign of personal weakness or a condition that can be willed or wished away. People who have a depressive illness cannot merely "pull themselves together" and get better. Without treatment, symptoms can last for

- Why do you worry unnecessarily? Who is it that you fear? Who can kill you? The soul is immortal.

- Whatever has happened has been good. Whatever is happening is good. Whatever will happen will be good. Do not regret the past. Do not worry about the future.

- What is it that you have lost? What did you bring that you have lost? What did you create that is now no more? You did not bring anything to this world. Whatever you took, you took here. You came empty-handed, and you will go empty-handed. Whatever belongs to you today belonged to someone else yesterday and will belong to someone else tomorrow. The cause of your misery is the illusory happiness that you derive by thinking about the things you own.

- Change is a rule of nature. What you think is death is actually life. Remove mine and yours, small and big from your mind. Then everything is yours, and you are for everyone.

- This body does not belong to you, and neither do you belong to this body. This body is made of elements found in nature and will go back into nature.

- Whatever you do, do it with a sense of detachment without owning and then you will always feel free and happy.

Note: Adapted from Indian philosophy as described in *Bhagvad Gita*, the Holy Scripture of Hindus.

weeks, months, or years. Appropriate treatment, however, can help more than 80 percent of those who suffer from depression.

Depression is more than feeling sad after a loss or becoming down because of a hard time. Like heart disease or diabetes, depression is a serious medical illness. It affects your thoughts, feelings, actions, and health. But as with most other illnesses, depression can be treated.

Anyone can become depressed. Depression is caused by many things, including extreme stress or grief, medical illness, prescribed medications, alcohol or drug use, family history and genetics, and other psychiatric disorders.

Depression rarely goes away by itself. You need to take action to feel better. For people who are depressed, the hardest thing to do is to reach out for help, but it is also the first step towards getting better.

The following tips can help you:

○ Find the cause.

○ Talk to a professional.

○ Take care of yourself.

○ Take stock of your blessings.

○ Stay active.

○ Get help.

○ Give it time.

Depressed? Have you lost interest in activities that used to bring you pleasure? Do you feel down, sad, or blue? Do you have trouble sleeping? Do you have headaches or other unexplained aches and pains? Have you gained or lost weight? Are you using drugs or alcohol to help you feel better? Everyone feels sad or blue some of the time, but if you have had these feelings for more than two weeks, it is time to seek help.

coping mechanisms

The word *cope* is derived from the Latin word *colpus* meaning "to alter" and, as defined in *Webster's Dictionary*, it is typically used in the psychological paradigm to denote "dealing with and attempting to overcome problems and difficulties." According to the transactional model described by Lazarus and Folkman (1984), there are two broad mechanisms of **coping**: problem focused and emotion focused. The problem-focused mechanism is based more on one's capability to think and alter the environmental event or situation (stressor). Examples of this strategy include utilization of problem-solving skills, interpersonal conflict resolution, advice seeking, time management, goal setting, and information gathering about the cause of one's stress. Problem solving requires thinking through various solutions, evaluating the pros and cons of different solutions, and then implementing a solution that seems most advantageous to reduce the stress. The emotion-oriented mechanism focuses inward on altering the way one thinks or feels about a situation or an event (stressor). Examples of this strategy include denying the existence of the stressful situation, freely expressing emotions, avoiding the stressful situation, relaxation, seeking social support, exercising, making social comparisons, or maximizing the positive points of the situation. In this chapter and workbook, we have presented a combination of these approaches.

METHOD BASED ON RATIONAL EMOTIVE THERAPY

(David, Szentagotai, Lupu, & Cosman, 2008; Dryden & DiGiuseppe, 1990; Ellis, 1971, 1975a, 1975b, 1990; Ellis & Grieger, 1977; Ellis & Harper, 1961; Walen, DiGiuseppe, & Wessler, 1980).

We are constantly engaging in self-talk—that is, the internal thought language by which we describe and interpret the world around us. If the beliefs of our self-talk are in consonance with reality, then we function well. If the beliefs are irrational and untrue, then they cause stress and emotional disturbance. Ellis's method of **rational emotive therapy** (RET) essentially challenges or refutes this very irrational thinking.

In RET, to be rational, we must be (a) practical, (b) logical, (c) objective, and (d) reality-based. On this basis, *rationality* is an attribute that helps us achieve our basic goals and purposes in life, to be logical, and to be consistently aware of reality. On the other hand, *irrationality* prevents us from achieving our basic goals and purposes, is illogical (especially dogmatic), and is inconsistent with reality. Based upon RET, some classical irrational ideas are depicted in Thoughts for Reflection 6.2, Rational Emotive Therapy's 11 Irrational Ideas (page 129).

The method based upon RET is popularly known as the ABCDE technique and consists of five steps:

A. *Activating System* The activating system may be either external or internal events that we face. It also includes inferences or interpretations about events around us.

B. *Belief System* The belief system consists of evaluative ideas or constructed views about the world around us.

C. *Consequences* Our beliefs have emotional and behavioral consequences. If our beliefs about negative activating events are rigid and irrational, then they result in disturbance and are termed *inappropriate negative consequences*. However, if our beliefs about negative activating events are flexible and rational, then they do not result in any disturbance and are termed *appropriate negative consequences*.

D. *Dispute Irrational Beliefs* Disputing irrational beliefs is the key component needed in order for this method to be effective. If we dispute the irrational beliefs in our mind, then we can also reduce the negative consequences that result. Examples of irrational beliefs include thinking that everyone will love you, thinking that you are competent in all respects, or thinking that all people are evil. Other irrational beliefs might be that it will be disastrous if things do not happen the way that you planned them or that happiness is completely controlled externally.

E. *Effect* As a result of disputing the irrational beliefs in our mind, we experience a new and more desirable consequence, which is referred to as the effect in this method.

Our ideas and beliefs may either be rigid or flexible. When these beliefs become rigid, they are usually irrational and take the form of "musts," "shoulds," "have tos," "got tos," and so on. These beliefs express themselves as:

○ "Awfulizing"—that is, classifying any situation as 100 percent bad

○ "I can't stand it"—that is, low frustration tolerance

○ "Damnation"—that is, being excessively critical of self, others, and/or life conditions

○ "Always" and "Never" thinking—that is, usage of extreme terms

When our beliefs are flexible, they are rational. These beliefs often take the form of desires, wishes, wants, and preferences. These rational beliefs express themselves as:

○ Moderate evaluations of badness—for example, "It is bad but not terrible."

○ Statements of tolerance—for example, "I don't like it, but I can bear it."

○ Acceptance of fallibility—for example, "I was wrong."

○ Avoidance of extremes—for example, "Often I do well" (instead of "I always do well").

You may now work through these steps using **Worksheet 6.2** (page 139)

METHOD BASED ON SIMPLIFIED KUNDALINI YOGA (SKY)

(Maharishi, 1989)

The **simplified kundalini yoga** (SKY) method, derived from Indian philosophy, is based on the principles of introspection as advocated by Yogiraj Vethathiri Maharishi, a contemporary philosopher and teacher from India who has formed the World Community Service Center, which has branches all over the world (see Chapter 3). This method entails the following steps:

Step 1. We need to seek a quiet place, have available at least one-half hour of uninterrupted time, and have a sheet of paper and pencil with us.

Step 2. We think, contemplate, and compile a list of all the worries that are bothering us at the present time.

Step 3. We classify the worries into four types:

a. *Worries to Be Faced* In this category worries such as chronic diseases, loss of property, and death will be listed. For example, a child is born with a birth defect (congenital anomaly). Despite all the best efforts, the child cannot be cured by medicine or other means. How can we solve this worry? What is the use of brooding over such a worry? To manage such worries, we need to resolve to be aware that there is no use worrying about things over which we have no control. Make your mind firm and abide by this resolution.

b. *Worries to Be Solved Immediately* Some worries have to be dealt with immediately and boldly. For example, one such worry is about general illness. It can be managed immediately by resorting to proper medication, diet, and lifestyle changes. Similarly, worries can arise out of differences of opinion in the family. We cannot disown our families; therefore, these worries need to be managed by mutual discussion without any delay. Worries about poverty and debts can be managed by hard work, perseverance, and changes in spending habits.

c. *Worries to Be Postponed* For example, consider a person who has reached an age suitable for marriage and is not able to find the right partner. For tackling such a worry, he or she has to keep trying patiently to find a mate and allow time to take its course. Therefore, action on such a worry can be postponed.

d. *Worries to Be Ignored* For example, our boss has a habit of constantly nagging us with outmoded ideas and notions. The best thing to do in such a situation would be to quietly keep on doing our best, unmindful of the purposeless advice given to us. This category involves worries arising out of differences of opinion, jealousy, and the like.

Step 4. Having classified all our worries into four types, the total number of worries to be tackled at the present time will be reduced. An unnecessary burden on our mind will be eased. Do not think that there will be no more worries in the future or that these worries will completely cease to exist. After one worry is resolved, another will "spring up." After we climb one mountain, another peak will come into our vision to be conquered. But what we can do now is work in a planned way to reduce our worries. **Worksheet 6.3** (page 141) helps you classify your worries according to this method in order to lessen the burden on your mind.

METHOD BASED ON GESTALT THERAPY

(Corey, 1991; Corsini & Wedding, 1995; Perls, 1969; Tonnesvang, Sommer, Hammink, & Sonne, 2010)

Gestalt is a German word meaning "whole" or "configuration" (Simkin, 1976). As one psychological dictionary puts it, Gestalt is "an integration of the whole as contrasted with summation of parts" (Warren, 1934). The originator of Gestalt therapy, Fredrick S. Perls, drew an analogy of the concept of this theory based on an organism that always works as a whole. Organisms are not a summation of parts but a coordination of organ systems or other components (Perls, 1969). **Gestalt therapy** emphasizes the unity of self-awareness, behavior, and experience. The goal of Gestalt therapy is to help us get in touch with reality and focus on the "now." It implicitly asks individuals to accept that they will be more comfortable and effective in their lives in the long run if they are fully aware of what they are doing from moment to moment and accept responsibility for their behaviors. By discovering *what is* rather than *what should be* or *what could have been,* or *the ideal of what should be or may be,* the person learns to trust himself or herself. A Gestalt prayer summarizes this philosophy (Perls, 1969):

> *I do my thing, and you do your thing.*
> *I am not in this world to live up to your expectations*
> *And you are not in this world to live up to mine.*
> *You are you, and I am I,*
> *And if by chance we find each other, it's beautiful.*
> *If not, it can't be helped.*

A modified process based on the principles of Gestalt therapy is provided in **Worksheet 6.4** (page 142) for you to practice.

SYSTEMATIC DESENSITIZATION

The **systematic densensitization** technique, first described by Joseph Wolpe (1958, 1973), involves imagining or experiencing an anxiety-provoking scene while practicing a response incompatible with anxiety (such as relaxation). This concept is also utilized in the field of medicine for treating allergies. The allergic patient is exposed to very small doses of allergen that are gradually increased until the body learns to accept the allergen. In coping with anxiety, the basic method entails slow and steady adjustments to small components of any problem. Each small step is considered one at a time, and relaxation is practiced alongside to counteract the adverse response. This technique involves developing a fear hierarchy, which is a sequence of small steps that lead to the anxiety-provoking event. Consider an example. Suppose we are students, and we have test anxiety. Our fear hierarchy would be as follows:

1. Enrolling for the course

2. Going to the classes

3. Completing the assignments

4. Studying the textbook

5. Studying additional materials

6. Reviewing the text

7. Preparing for examinations

8. Going to the examination

9. Waiting before the examination

10. Taking the examination

11. Waiting for the results of the examination

12. Obtaining the results

Most of the test anxiety is tied into the *expectations* of obtaining a good result, and therefore we have included that dimension in the fear hierarchy. Similarly, we can construct a fear hierarchy for any fear that causes us anxiety. This procedure has been described systematically in a step-by-step fashion in **Worksheet 6.5** (page 144) for you to practice.

You should practice the techniques described in this chapter and find the one that is best for you. Keep practicing that technique to obtain the best results. You may want to change from one technique to another over time, or you may want to practice the same technique. The approach will vary from one person to another.

See Box 6.2, Emotional Intelligence (page 133), for a discussion of the ability to use emotions to solve problems.

BOX **6·2**

Emotional Intelligence

In recent years, a school of thought in psychological research has emerged emphasizing that the role of emotional maturity is as important or even more important than intelligence for success in academics and life. Partly, this concept has emerged because, while intelligence quotient (IQ) does predict academic achievement and occupational status, it is able to account for only 10 to 20 percent of the personal variation in these areas. The other developments that have contributed to greater interest in this line of thought include a popular book by Daniel Goleman (1995) on the subject, coverage of this concept in some popular television talk shows, and some empirical research (Mayer & Salovey, 1997). Emotional intelligence has been defined as the ability to use emotions to solve problems. Five primary components of emotional intelligence have been identified (Goleman, 1995):

1. *Self-awareness* involves knowing one's emotions, recognizing feelings as they occur, and discriminating between them.

2. *Mood management* entails handling feelings so that they become relevant to the current situation and reacting appropriately.

3. *Self-motivation* includes "gathering up" one's feelings and directing oneself toward a goal, despite self-doubt, inertia, and impulsiveness.

4. *Empathy* is the ability to recognize feelings in others and tune into their verbal and nonverbal cues.

5. *Managing relationships* requires handling interpersonal interaction, conflict resolution, and negotiations.

Research continues in refining these constructs, measuring these attributes, and ascertaining their contribution and applicability in various facets of life. For the reader in stress management, it would be worthwhile to explore the role of each of these dimensions for anxiety reduction in particular. The major shift required for transcribing this concept is the focus on one's emotions rather than cognitive abilities. While there is indeed an overlap between cognition (thinking) and emotions, perhaps a greater awareness of the latter can enhance one's effectiveness. In simple terms, the following five steps would be helpful in this endeavor:

- Recognizing feelings in oneself
- Recognizing feelings in others
- Caring for others' feelings
- Regulating feelings in oneself
- Harnessing feelings to improving relationships

CHAPTER REVIEW

summary points

○ Anxiety arises out of inefficiency and fear.

○ Excessive anxiety is associated with generalized anxiety disorder and panic disorder.

○ The Taylor Manifest Anxiety Scale measures trait anxiety.

○ The rational emotive therapy (RET)-based ABCDE technique described by Albert Ellis consists of five steps: identifying the activating system, identifying the belief system, identifying the consequences, disputing irrational beliefs, and visualizing the effects.

- Coping with anxiety using simplified kundalini yoga (SKY), as described by Yogiraj Vethathiri Maharishi, consists of classifying worries into those to be faced, those to be solved immediately, those to be postponed, and those to be ignored.

- Coping with anxiety using Gestalt therapy described by Fredrick Perls helps us to focus on the "now," discovering "what is reality," and bearing the pain, if any.

- Systematic desensitization described by Joseph Wolpe involves analyzing any anxiety-provoking situation in terms of smaller steps and counteracting those steps at each stage by practicing relaxation.

important terms defined

anxiety: A state of mind that perceives the outside event or one's action as resulting in negative outcomes and one's lack of ability to cope.

coping: The ability to deal with and overcome problems and difficulties encountered in life.

Gestalt therapy: A comprehensive coping technique in which the person learns to focus on present and total reality.

rational emotive therapy: A self-analysis coping process based on logical, practical, objective, reality-based appraisal of stressors. *See also* **coping**.

simplified kundalini yoga: A set of meditation techniques designed to enhance harmony between body, mind, and environment.

state anxiety: Anxiety due to being in a given stressful situation. *See also* **anxiety; trait anxiety**.

systematic desensitization: A coping method designed to overcome anxiety-provoking events based on breaking down the complex set of events into small steps as fear hierarchy. *See also* **anxiety**.

trait anxiety: Anxiety due to one's personality disposition. *See also* **anxiety; state anxiety**.

websites to explore

ANXIETY AND DEPRESSION ASSOCIATION OF AMERICA

www.adaa.org

The ADAA website provides information about dealing with anxiety disorders. The ADAA provides information, links to treatment providers, and helpful information for dealing with stress.

- Explore the information about "College Students" under the "Living and Thriving" tab. How would you help yourself or a friend deal with an anxiety disorder?

MATH ANXIETY

www.mathacademy.com/pr/minitext/anxiety/index.asp

Math anxiety is very common among students. This website defines math anxiety, delineates math myths, and provides practical tips to overcome math anxiety.

- Review and apply these tips if you suffer from math anxiety.

PSYCHOTHERAPY FOR POSTTRAUMATIC STRESS DISORDER (PTSD)

http://ptsd.factsforhealth.org/anxiety.html

This website provides specific information about breathing training, relaxation, assertiveness, positive thinking/self-talk, and thought stopping in combating PTSD.

▧ Review the website and the links. What is PTSD? How will you help a person suffering from PTSD?

MENTAL HEALTH: A REPORT OF THE SURGEON GENERAL

http://profiles.nlm.nih.gov/ps/retrieve/ResourceMetadata/NNBBHS

This website presents the Mental Health: A Report of the Surgeon General, published in 1999.

▧ Read the summary and, if possible, the entire report. Prepare a brief reaction paper.

TEST ANXIETY

www.testanxietytips.com/

Most students feel anxiety while taking tests. This website provides information and practical tips for dealing with test anxiety.

▧ Review the approach described on this website. How will you go about incorporating it into your life?

Taylor Manifest Anxiety Scale

Indicate whether each item is true or false for you.

_____ 1. I do not tire quickly.

_____ 2. I am troubled by attacks of nausea.

_____ 3. I believe I am no more nervous than most others.

_____ 4. I have very few headaches.

_____ 5. I work under a great deal of tension.

_____ 6 I cannot keep my mind on one thing.

_____ 7. I worry over money and business.

_____ 8. I frequently notice that my hand shakes when I try to do something.

_____ 9. I blush no more often than others do.

_____ 10. I have diarrhea once a month or more.

_____ 11. I worry quite a bit over possible misfortunes.

_____ 12. I practically never blush.

_____ 13. I am often afraid that I am going to blush.

_____ 14. I have nightmares every few nights.

_____ 15. My hands and feet are usually warm enough.

_____ 16. I sweat very easily, even on cool days.

_____ 17. Sometimes when embarrassed, I break out in a sweat, which annoys me greatly.

_____ 18. I hardly ever notice my heart pounding, and I am seldom short of breath.

_____ 19. I feel hungry almost all the time.

_____ 20. I am very seldom troubled by constipation.

_____ 21. I have a great deal of stomach trouble.

_____ 22. I have had periods in which I lost sleep over worry.

_____ 23. My sleep is fitful and disturbed.

_____ 24. I dream frequently about things that are best kept to myself.

_____ 25. I am easily embarrassed.

_____ 26. I am more sensitive than most other people.

Taylor Manifest Anxiety Scale (*cont'd*)

_____ 27. I frequently find myself worrying about something.

_____ 28. I wish I could be as happy as others seem to be.

_____ 29. I am usually calm and not easily upset.

_____ 30. I cry easily.

_____ 31. I feel anxiety about something or someone almost all the time.

_____ 32. I am happy most of the time.

_____ 33. It makes me nervous to have to wait.

_____ 34. I have periods of such great restlessness that I cannot sit long in a chair.

_____ 35. Sometimes I become so excited that I find it hard to get to sleep.

_____ 36. I have sometimes felt that difficulties were piling up so high that I could not overcome them.

_____ 37. I must admit that I have at times been worried beyond reason over something that really did not matter.

_____ 38. I have very few fears compared to my friends.

_____ 39. I have been afraid of things or people that I know could not hurt me.

_____ 40. I certainly feel useless at times.

_____ 41. I find it hard to keep my mind on a task or job.

_____ 42. I am usually self-conscious.

_____ 43. I am inclined to take things hard.

_____ 44. I am a high-strung person.

_____ 45. Life is a strain for me much of the time.

_____ 46. At times I think I am no good at all.

_____ 47. I am certainly lacking in self-confidence.

_____ 48. I sometimes feel that I am about to go to pieces.

_____ 49. I shrink from facing a crisis or difficulty.

_____ 50. I am entirely self-confident.

_____

Note: From "A personality scale of manifest anxiety" by J. A. Taylor, 1953, *Journal of Abnormal and Social Psychology, 48*, 285–290. Copyright 1953 by Journal of Abnormal and Social Psychology.

FEEDBACK ON WORKSHEET 6.1

Give yourself one point for each of the following responses:

1. False	11. True	21. True	31. True	41. True
2. True	12. False	22. True	32. False	42. True
3. False	13. True	23. True	33. True	43. True
4. False	14. True	24. True	34. True	44. True
5. True	15. False	25. True	35. True	45. True
6. True	16. True	26. True	36. True	46. True
7. True	17. True	27. True	37. True	47. True
8. True	18. False	28. True	38. False	48. True
9. False	19. True	29. False	39. True	49. True
10. True	20. False	30. True	40. True	50. False

The average score on this scale is approximately 19. If you scored below 19, you feel less anxious than the average person, and if you scored above 19, you feel more anxious than the average person. If you scored over 35 on this scale, then your anxiety levels are very high, and you may need to seek professional consultation.

Anxiety Reduction through RET

Seek out a quiet place and put aside everything else that you have been doing. Now, follow the steps outlined below.

STEP 1. ACTIVATING SYSTEM

Write down the facts of a recent event at a time when you were upset. Include only objective facts, not conjectures, subjective impressions, or value judgments.

_____

_____

_____

_____

_____

STEP 2. BELIEF SYSTEM

Write down all your judgments, beliefs, assumptions, perceptions, and worries pertaining to the event of Step 1.

_____

_____

_____

_____

_____

STEP 3. CONSEQUENCES

Identify the physical, mental, and behavioral results of the event. Try to present these in the form of a summary word or words—for example, *anger, grief.*

_____

_____

_____

_____

_____

(continued)

Anxiety Reduction through RET *(cont'd)*

STEP 4. DISPUTE IRRATIONAL BELIEFS

a. Select one irrational belief at a time.

_____

_____

_____

_____

b. Is there any rational support for this idea? Your response needs to be no.

_____

_____

_____

_____

c. Assign reasons for this falseness.

_____

_____

_____

_____

d. What is the worst thing that can happen according to this irrational idea?

_____

_____

_____

_____

e. What are the good things that can happen if you do not accept this irrational idea?

_____

_____

_____

_____

STEP 5. EFFECT

Prepare for the worst events that can happen if you accept this irrational belief. Focus on the benefits that can occur if you do not accept this irrational belief. Give autosuggestions (self-talk) to refute this irrational belief. As a consequence of this new thinking, you will experience the positive results. Proceed in a similar fashion with other irrational ideas, and practice this technique regularly.

Anxiety Reduction through Simplified Kundalini Yoga (SKY) as taught by Yogiraj Vethathiri Maharishi

Seek out a quiet place for at least 30 minutes of contemplation. Think about what is on your mind and classify the issues into the following categories:

Issues to Be Faced	Issues to Be Tackled Immediately	Issues to Be Deferred for Tackling Later	Issues to Be Overlooked

Note: Based on *Yoga for modern age* (3rd ed.) by Y.V. Maharishi, 1989, Madras, India: Vethathiri Publications. Copyright 1989 by Y.V. Maharishi. Reprinted by permission.

FEEDBACK ON WORKSHEET 6.3

Classifying your worries into the four categories probably resulted in reducing the total number of worries to be tackled at the *present* time, as well as an unnecessary burden on your mind. Whenever your mind is flooded with a number of worries and problems, you can sit down and practice this technique to reduce the total number of worries at any time. This technique is a useful and effective approach that conserves energy for other productive activities.

Coping with Anxiety Based on Gestalt Therapy

Go through the following steps and write down your responses wherever needed.

Step 1. Seek out a quiet place and focus on your thinking.

Step 2. Write down all the thoughts that are coming into your mind. At the same time, be consciously aware of your body movements, if any.

Thoughts:

_____

_____

_____

_____

_____

_____

_____

_____

_____

_____

_____

_____

_____

_____

_____

_____

_____

_____

_____

Coping with Anxiety Based on Gestalt Therapy *(cont'd)*

Body movements/sensations during thoughts:

_____

_____

_____

_____

_____

Step 3. List the painful thoughts that you do not want to come into your mind.

_____

_____

_____

_____

_____

Step 4. Experience the pain associated with your thoughts with awareness rather than the need to alleviate it. If painful thoughts become too overbearing, then you should stop and relax.

FEEDBACK ON WORKSHEET 6.4

Try to establish consonance between your thoughts and your body movements. If you are not able to derive any inferences, do not worry—just proceed. Practice this awareness-building exercise and *always focus on now*—that is, on the thoughts that are arising at this moment in time. If painful thoughts become too overbearing, then you should stop and relax. This method can be practiced individually or in groups. With regular practice, your skills in coping with anxiety will improve.

Systematic Desensitization

You should proceed according to the following steps.

Step 1. Seek a quiet, comfortable, and peaceful place. Select a relaxation technique described in Chapter 3 and relax. Write down the name of this technique:

_____

Print the word "relax":

_____

Step 2. Now you should develop a fear hierarchy for the fear that causes you anxiety. Write down all the small steps leading to that fear. You should try to come up with a minimum of 10 steps.

Fear: _____

Hierarchy:

a. _____

b. _____

c. _____

d. _____

e. _____

f. _____

g. _____

h. _____

i. _____

j. _____

Step 3. Relax.

Step 4. Imagine the first item in the fear hierarchy list for 1 to 5 seconds. Gradually increase the thinking time to **about 1 minute.**

Step 5. Relax.

Step 6. Repeat Step 4 on the next item. If you have difficulty with any item, break it down further into smaller steps and approach it gradually in your mind. You need to reassure yourself that there is nothing to fear.

FEEDBACK ON WORKSHEET 6.5

With regular practice of this technique, you will be able to get over your fear and reduce anxiety when you encounter that event. In this way, you will be able to strengthen your mind and not be bogged down by small fears.

references and further readings

Allen, R. J., & Hyde, D. (1980). *Investigations in stress control.* Minneapolis: Burgess.

Chou, S. P., Lee, H. K., Cho, M. J., Park, J. I., Dawson, D. A., Grant, B. F. (2011). Alcohol use disorders, nicotine dependence, and co-occurring mood and anxiety disorders in the United States and South Korea-A cross-national comparison. *Alcoholism, Clinical and Experimental Research,* doi: 10.1111/j.1530-0277.2011.01639.x

Corey, G. (1991). *Theory and practice of counseling and psychotherapy.* Pacific Grove, CA: Brooks/Cole.

Corsini, R. J., & Wedding, D. (1995). *Current psychotherapies* (5th ed.). Itasca, IL: Peacock.

Culpepper, L. (2002). Generalized anxiety disorders in primary care: Emerging issues in management and treatment. *Journal of Clinical Psychiatry, 63* (Suppl. 8), 35–42.

David, D., Szentagotai, A., Lupu, V., & Cosman, D. (2008). Rational emotive behavior therapy, cognitive therapy, and medication in the treatment of major depressive disorder: A randomized clinical trial, post treatment outcomes, and six-month follow-up. *Journal of Clinical Psychology, 64*(6), 728–746.

Diagnostic and statistical manual of mental disorders (4th ed. text rev.). (DSM IV-TR). (2000). Washington, DC: American Psychiatric Association.

Dryden, W., & DiGiuseppe, R. (1990). *A primer on rational emotive therapy.* Champaign, IL: Research Press.

Ellis, A. (1971). *Growth through reason.* Palo Alto, CA: Science & Behavior.

Ellis, A. (1975a). *A new guide to rational living.* North Hollywood, CA: Wilshire.

Ellis, A. (1975b). *How to live with a neurotic at home and at work* (rev. ed.). North Hollywood, CA: Wilshire.

Ellis, A. (1990). *How to stubbornly refuse to make yourself miserable about anything—yes, anything.* New York: Carol.

Ellis, A., & Grieger, R. (1977). *RET handbook of rational emotive therapy.* New York: Springer.

Ellis, A., & Harper, R. (1961). *A guide to rational living.* North Hollywood, CA: Wilshire.

Goleman, D. (1995). *Emotional intelligence: Why it can matter more than IQ for character, health and lifelong achievement.* New York: Bantam.

Greenberg, J. S. (2010). *Comprehensive stress management* (12th ed.). Boston: McGraw-Hill.

Kessler, R. C., & Wittchow, H. U. (2002). Patterns and correlates of generalized anxiety disorders in community samples. *Journal of Clinical Psychiatry, 63* (Suppl. 8), 4–10.

Lazarus, R. S., & Folkman, S. (1984). *Stress, appraisal and coping.* New York: Springer.

Maharishi, Y. V. (1989). *Yoga for modern age* (3rd ed.). Madras, India: Vethathiri.

Mayer, J. D., & Salovey, P. (1997). What is emotional intelligence? In P. Salovey & D. Sluyter (Eds.), *Emotional development, emotional literacy and emotional intelligence.* New York: Basic Books.

Perls, F. S. (1969). *Gestalt therapy verbatim.* Moab, UT: Real People Press.

Piero, A. (2010). Personality correlates of impulsivity in subjects with generalized anxiety disorders. *Comprehensive Psychiatry, 51*(5), 538–545.

Regier, D. A., Boyd, J. H., Burke, J. D., Jr., et al. (1988). One month prevalence of mental disorders in the United States: Based on five epidemiological catchment area sites. *Archives of General Psychiatry, 45,* 977–986.

Shader, R. I., & Greenblatt, D. J. (1993). Use of benzodiazepines in anxiety disorders. *New England Journal of Medicine, 328*, 1398–1405.

Simkin, J. S. (1976). *Gestalt therapy: Mini lectures.* Millbrae, CA: Celestial Arts.

Taylor, J. A. (1953). A personality scale of manifest anxiety. *Journal of Abnormal and Social Psychology, 48,* 285–290.

Tonnesvang, J., Sommer, U., Hammink, J., Sonne, M. (2010). Gestalt therapy and cognitive therapy—Contrasts or complementarities? *Psychotherapy, 47*(4), 586–602.

Walen, S. R., DiGiuseppe, R., & Wessler, R. L. (1980). *A practitioner's guide to rational emotive therapy.* New York: Oxford University Press.

Warren, H. D. (1934). *Dictionary of Psychology.* New York: Houghton Mifflin.

Wolpe, J. (1958). *Psychotherapy by reciprocal inhibition.* Stanford, CA: Stanford University Press.

Wolpe, J. (1973). *The practice of behavior therapy* (2nd ed.). New York: Pergamon.

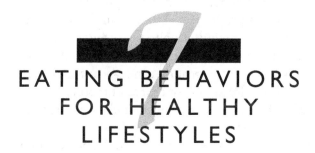

EATING BEHAVIORS FOR HEALTHY LIFESTYLES

Enjoy balanced meals at regular times, and cherish the gift.

importance of appropriate eating

In a classical study, Belloc and Breslow (1972), after surveying nearly 7,000 individuals, identified seven behaviors related to the maintenance of personal health:

1. Sleeping 7 to 8 hours daily

2. Eating breakfast almost daily

3. Consuming planned snacks

4. Being at or near prescribed weight

5. Never smoking cigarettes

6. Moderate or no use of alcohol

7. Regular physical activity

The exact role and mechanism of each of the above factors are not completely understood, but it has generally been accepted that all these factors contribute significantly toward maintaining health and longevity. In this chapter we primarily focus on eating behaviors for healthy lifestyles. The importance of eating nutritious meals appropriately plays a significant role in healthy living, helps combat daily stress, and also reduces undue stress. Though the relationship between diet and stress has not been studied extensively (Greenberg, 2010), the importance of eating appropriately to maintain health and reduce stress cannot be ruled out (Girdano, Everly, & Dusek, 2012). Healthy eating enhances coping abilities against various stressors and stressful events. When meals consist of all the ingredients of a balanced diet, then the body has sufficient energy to cope with stress. A balanced diet also provides enough reserves to manage stress.

Irregular eating of meals, eating improper food (that is, undercooked or overcooked, too spicy or too bland, consisting of only one category of food, stale, unpalatable, and so on), undereating, or overeating unduly taxes the body and is a potential source of stress in itself. Overeating can lead to being overweight and obese. Overweight and obesity are major causes of mortality in the United States and most industrialized countries of the world. In the United States, the prevalence of obesity has been increasing since the 1980s (Flegal, Carroll, Kuczmarski, & Johnson, 1998). According to the National Health and Nutrition Examination Survey (NHANES), the prevalence of obesity is 35.5 percent in adult men and 35.8 percent in adult women (Flegal, Carroll, Kit, & Ogden, 2012). The age-adjusted mean Body Mass Index (BMI) in this survey was 28.7 for both men and women. Overweight is defined as BMI greater than or equal to 25 kg/m^2 and obesity as BMI greater than or equal to 30 kg/m^2.

If we eat balanced, healthy meals after sufficient appetite has set in and do not indulge in overeating, then the body is saved from undue stress and associated negative consequences. However, undereating also creates stress for the body because not enough energy is available to perform daily activities. Therefore, the key lies in maintaining a *balance* of quantity and quality of food and regularity in eating. The United States Department of Agriculture (USDA) has given *Dietary Guidelines for Americans, 2010* (USDA, 2012) which suggests the following key recommendations for the general population. (Note: The *Dietary Guidelines for Americans, 2010* is available at www.cnpp.usda.gov/ DietaryGuidelines.htm.)

DIETARY GUIDELINES FOR AMERICANS, 2010

Balancing Calories to Manage Weight

○ Prevent and/or reduce overweight/obesity through improved eating behaviors and physical activity behaviors.

○ Control total caloric intake to manage body weight. For overweight and obese people this implies taking less calories from food and beverages.

○ Increase physical activity.

○ For each stage of life, choose appropriate caloric intake.

Foods to Reduce

○ Reduce daily sodium intake to less than 2,300 mg. For African Americans, those over 51 years, those who have hypertension, kidney disease, or diabetes, the goal is to reduce sodium intake to less than 1,500 mg.

○ Consume less than 10 percent of calories from saturated fatty acids by replacing them with monounsaturated and polyunsaturated fatty acids.

○ Consume less than 300 mg of dietary cholesterol.

○ Keep *trans* fatty acid consumption to a minimum by limiting foods that contain synthetic sources of *trans* fats, such as partially hydrogenated oils, and by limiting other solid fats.

○ Reduce the intake of calories from solid fats and added sugars.

○ Limit the consumption of refined grains.

○ If one drinks alcohol, drinking should be in moderation: a maximum of one drink per day for women and two drinks per day for men who are of legal age.

Foods to Increase

○ Increase fruit and vegetable consumption.

○ Eat a variety of vegetables, especially dark-green, red and orange vegetables and beans and peas.

○ Consume at least half of all grains as whole grains. Increase whole-grain intake by replacing refined grains with whole grains.

○ Increase intake of fat-free or low-fat milk and milk products, such as milk, yogurt, cheese, or fortified soy beverages.

○ Choose a variety of protein foods, which include seafood, lean meat and poultry, eggs, beans and peas, soy products, and unsalted nuts and seeds.

○ Increase the amount and variety of seafood consumed by choosing seafood in place of some meat and poultry.

○ Replace protein foods that are higher in solid fats with choices that are lower in solid fats and calories and/or are sources of oils.

○ Use oils to replace solid fats where possible.

○ Choose foods that provide more potassium, dietary fiber, calcium, and vitamin D. These foods include vegetables, fruits, whole grains, and milk and milk products.

Recommendations for Women Capable of Becoming Pregnant

○ Choose foods that supply heme iron, which is more readily absorbed by the body, additional iron sources, and enhancers of iron absorption such as vitamin C-rich foods.

○ Consume 400 micrograms (mcg) per day of synthetic folic acid (from fortified foods and/or supplements) in addition to food forms of folate from the diet.

Recommendations for Pregnant and Breast Feeding Women

○ Consume 8 to 12 ounces of seafood per week from a variety of seafood types.

○ Limit tuna to 6 ounces per week and do not eat the following four types of fish: tilefish, shark, swordfish, and king mackerel.

○ Take an iron supplement, if pregnant.

❍ Select an eating pattern that meets nutrient needs over time at an appropriate calorie level.

❍ Account for all foods and beverages consumed and assess how they fit within a total healthy eating pattern.

❍ Follow food safety recommendations when preparing and eating foods to reduce the risk of foodborne illnesses.

DISORDERED EATING AND BODY IMAGE

When we eat right, our body is able to deal with stress effectively. When we do not eat right, the effects of stress on the body increase. Sometimes, eating improperly can also lead to eating disorders. One such disorder is *anorexia nervosa*, which is characterized by significant weight loss resulting from excessive food restriction. Another disorder is *bulimia nervosa*, which is characterized by a cycle of binge eating followed by purging or excessive physical activity to try and rid the body of unwanted calories. A variant of bulimia is *binge eating disorder*, which is characterized by consuming large quantities of food in a very short period of time until the individual is uncomfortably full. Binge eating is not accompanied by purging. Finally, there is *compulsive overeating*, which is characterized by uncontrollable eating and consequent weight gain. Most people suffering from eating disorders use food as a way to cope with stress, emotional conflicts, and daily problems. One should strive to eat right so that eating disorders do not occur.

Another source of stress can arise from our body image. Body image is often influenced by the media. The media presents physical images that are almost flawless, and we want those images for ourselves. The reality is that no one looks "perfect" naturally—not even the models portrayed in the media. The media tries to sell these images to us with the message that if we try hard, we can have the look we want and shaping our body will somehow bring us success and happiness. This is not true. We have learned how to maintain a healthy weight, but it is not healthy to be obsessed by the way we look. We must make a genuine effort to eat right to maintain our weight and be satisfied with the way we look.

enhancing awareness
about our dietary patterns

How well do we eat? Is our diet balanced? Do we eat our meals regularly? These are some of the questions that we may not be able to answer impromptu. The reason is that most of us seldom take time to think about what we eat and how we eat. We have taken eating for granted. We need to become more aware of our diet and eating patterns and consider a change. Awareness about our diet and eating patterns is a central and important step in effecting a change in our behavior. Therefore, before you proceed any further, become more aware of your own dietary habits and patterns with the help of **Worksheet 7.1** on page 163.

categories of food items

Let's briefly understand the various types of food items and what they do to our body. The various food items can be classified, from a nutrition point of view, into the following six categories:

1. ***Carbohydrates*** Carbohydrate is a word from chemistry. The word *carbohydrate* is derived from *carbo*, implying "carbon," and *hydrate*, implying "hydrogen and oxygen." That is, these compounds constitute various proportions of carbon, hydrogen, and oxygen. Food items rich in carbohydrates include sugars, bread (wheat flour), the fibrous portions of fruits and vegetables, cereals, rice, pasta (wheat flour), roots and tubers, and so on. These food items, when consumed and digested, provide the body with energy. This energy helps the body perform its daily activities. They also provide the body with fiber, which helps decrease elevated **cholesterol** and blood glucose levels. Fiber is "filling" and so helps with weight control and also adds to the bulk that facilitates easy elimination from the bowel.

   It is important to consume this vital category of food in moderation. If too little carbohydrates are consumed, then the body does not get enough energy to perform daily tasks. If carbohydrates are ingested in excess, the body tends to convert and store these products, often as fat, for future use. If this excess carbohydrate ingestion persists for a long time and is at the cost of other vital food items, then fat deposition and other health-related problems occur. Further, if our diet solely consists of carbohydrates, then the body is deprived of other vital categories of food items, and the body is weakened, especially in coping with long-term demands of stress. Thus, the importance of using moderation and combining this category with other food categories cannot be overemphasized.

   Determining the correct amount of carbohydrates to be consumed depends on many factors, including the amount of daily activity, type of activities, body constitution, and so on. MyPlate, shown in Figure 7.1, below, shows that grains should be one-fourth of the eating plate. If our activity levels are more sedentary in nature or if our body constitution is smaller, we may stick

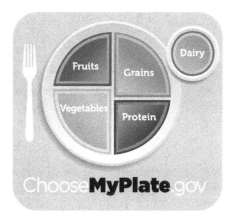

Note: From the U.S. Department of Agriculture (USDA) Center for Nutrition Policy and Promotion. www.cnpp.usda.gov/MyPlate.htm

Figure 7.1 MyPlate

At the Supermarket

■ Read ingredient labels. Identify added sugars in a product, and select items lower in added sugars when possible. A food is likely to be high in sugars if one of these names appears first or second in the ingredient list or if several names are listed:

brown sugar	invert sugar
corn sweetener	lactose
corn syrup	malt syrup
dextrose	maltose
fructose	molasses
fruit juice concentrate	raw sugar
glucose	sucrose

■ Buy fresh fruits or fruits packed in water or juice, rather than those in light or heavy syrup.

■ Buy fewer foods that are high in sugars, such as presweetened cereals, soft drinks, fruit-flavored punches, and sweet desserts. Be aware that some low-fat desserts may be very high in sugars.

In the Kitchen

■ Reduce the sugars in foods you prepare at home. Try new recipes or make your own. Start by reducing sugars gradually until you have decreased them by one-third or more.

■ Experiment with spices such as cinnamon, cardamom, coriander, nutmeg, ginger, and mace to enhance the sweet flavor of foods. Spiced foods will taste sweeter if warmed.

■ When possible, use home-prepared items (made with less sugar) instead of commercially prepared ones that are higher in sugar.

At the Table

■ Use less of all sugars, including white and brown sugars, honey, molasses, syrups, jams, and jellies.

■ Choose fewer foods that are high in added sugars, such as prepared baked goods, candies, and sweet desserts.

■ Reach for fresh fruit instead of something sweetened with additional sugars for dessert or a snack.

■ Add less sugar to foods—coffee, tea, cereal, or fruit. Get used to using half as much sugar, then see if you can cut back even more.

■ Cut back on the number of sugar-sweetened soft drinks, punches, lemonade and limeade you drink.

Note: From *Use sugars only in moderation* (P. 5) by U.S. Department of Agriculture (Human Nutrition Information Service), July 1993, Washington DC: Government Printing Office; and *Nutrition and your health: Dietary guidelines for Americans, 2005,* by U.S. Department of Agriculture, 2005, Washington, DC: Public Health Service. For more tips, go to www.choosemyplate.gov.

to the lower limit of the carbohydrates for observing moderation. The *Dietary Guidelines for Americans, 2010* (USDA, 2012) recommends that half of your grain choices come from whole grains. Use of sugars needs to be curtailed; Thoughts for Reflection 7.1, Using Sugars in Moderation—Some Suggestions, above, provides some suggestions.

2. **Proteins** The word *protein* is derived from the Greek word *proteios,* meaning "prime" or "chief." Proteins are in fact the most important constituents of our diet. There are two major sources of dietary proteins: (a) *animal sources*: eggs, milk, meat, fish, and so on; and (b) *plant sources*: lentils, cereals, nuts, beans, and so on. The prime function of protein is as a *building block*. Proteins are needed for growth, maintenance, and replacement of body cells. They are also required in the production of most hormones and enzymes, which regulate body functions. To combat stress, proteins are important constituents. If the diet lacks

enough proteins, then the body becomes emaciated, and stress-fighting capabilities are also substantially reduced. Extreme environmental or physiological stresses increase nitrogen loss through urine and increase energy expenditure (Cuthberston, 1964). This effect necessitates the need for greater amounts of protein intake. However, if the diet contains excess protein, then it is converted to fat and stored for future use. If this excess persists, it is also not good for the body. It may lead to unwanted and unused by-products, which are potentially harmful. Some proteins are also responsible for allergic manifestations in many susceptible people. Therefore, *moderation* of protein intake is essential. Again, choice is important. We want to decrease intake of meats high in saturated fats and increase intake of fish (rich in omega-3 fatty acids); choose lean poultry, beef, and pork cuts; and increase intake of legumes, nuts, and soy. MyPlate recommends that a little less than one-fourth of the eating plate must be proteins.

3. **Fats** Fats are sources of energy and are important in helping transport some vitamins (fat-soluble vitamins). They also add flavor to foods. Dietary fats are derived from two sources: (a) *animal sources*: butter, lard, and so on; and (b) *plant sources*: various edible oils such as sunflower, canola, olive, and so on. Research demonstrates positive health benefits of consuming monounsaturated fats, omega-3 fats, and some polyunsaturated fatty acids (benefits include lower inflammation and lower low-density lipoprotein cholesterol). Fats should be used moderately in the diet. The newest dietary recommendations from the National Academy of Sciences (2002) are 45 to 65 percent of calories from carbohydrates, 20 to 35 percent of calories from fat, and 10 to 35 percent of calories from protein. (Persons who have metabolic syndrome do better with more fat and less carbohydrates.) As explained earlier, the body requires small quantities of fat to perform some vital functions. However, when taken in excess, they tend to accumulate in the body. Excess deposition of fats leads to obesity, which has been associated as a risk factor for a number of disorders, including coronary heart disease and stroke. Thoughts for Reflection 7.2, Easy Ways to Cut Fat, Saturated Fat, and Cholesterol in Your Diet (page 154), provides some suggestions for reducing cholesterol and fats in the diet.

4. **Vitamins** The word *vitamin* is derived from the earlier German word *vitamine* (*vita,* meaning "life," and *amine,* based on the earlier notion that all these substances contained amino acids chemically). Vitamins are substances that are needed by the body in extremely small amounts. Though vitamins do not supply energy directly, they do help in the release of energy from other substances and play an important role in many chemical reactions within the body. Vitamins can be broadly classified into two types: (a) *fat soluble*: A, D, E, and K; and (b) *water soluble*: B and C. Some of the key sources of vitamins are depicted in Table 7.1 (page 155).

If fat-soluble vitamins are consumed in excess, they tend to accumulate in the body. This accumulation is responsible for a disorder called *hypervitaminosis.* There is consensus that these vitamins should not be taken in excess as supplements. Water-soluble vitamins, if taken in excess, are easily excreted out of the system. However, authorities are divided on recommending their excess use. Some believe they cause no harm, but others believe that they can be harmful too (for example, taking excess vitamin C can cause formation of renal stones). We recommend a balance in taking vitamins. From a stress

**EASY WAYS
TO CUT FAT,
SATURATED
FAT, AND
CHOLESTEROL
IN YOUR DIET**

At the Store

- Choose lean cuts of meat, such as beef round, loin, sirloin, arm or chuck roasts, and pork loin chops.

- Consider fish and poultry as alternatives; they are somewhat lower in saturated fat.

- Buy low-fat versions of dairy products.

- Read the food label and choose foods that are lower in fat, saturated fat, and cholesterol.

In the Kitchen

- When cooking, replace saturated fats, such as butter and lard, with small amounts of polyunsaturated and monounsaturated fats in vegetable oils such as corn oil, soybean oil, olive oil, peanut oil, or canola oil.

- Broil, roast, bake, steam, or boil foods instead of frying them, or try stir-frying with just a little fat.

- Trim all visible fat from meat before it is cooked. Remove skin from poultry.

- Spoon off fat from meat dishes after they are cooked.

- Use skim milk or low-fat milk when making cream sauces, soups, or puddings.

- Substitute low-fat yogurt or whipped low-fat cottage cheese for sour cream and mayonnaise in dips and dressings.

- Substitute two egg whites for each whole egg in recipes for most quick breads, cookies, and cakes. (Cholesterol and fat are in the yolk, not in the white.)

- Try lemon juice, herbs, or spices to season foods instead of butter or margarine.

At the Table

- Use less of *all* fats and oils, especially saturated fats such as butter, cream, sour cream, and cream cheese.

- Try reduced-calorie salad dressings— they are usually low in fat.

- As a beverage, gradually replace whole milk with 2-percent-fat milk, then 1-percent-fat or skim milk.

Note: From Food facts for older adults: Information on how to use the dietary guidelines (p. 6) by Human Nutrition Information Service, U.S. Department of Agriculture and National Institute on Aging, National Institutes of Health, 1993, Hyattsville, MD: U.S. Department of Agriculture.

management point of view, vitamins are essential in optimum quantities for maintaining the body's resistance to stress.

5. *Minerals* Minerals are also needed in relatively small amounts. Minerals are used to make hemoglobin in red blood cells and strengthen bones and teeth. They are also essential to maintain body fluids and chemical reactions in the body. They improve the body's ability to manage stress effectively if taken in optimum quantities. Some minerals that are helpful in combating stress are calcium, iron, zinc, selenium (potent antioxidant), and magnesium. The **electrolytes** of sodium, potassium, and chloride also need to be in balance to manage stress. It is important to reduce the intake of table salt (sodium chloride), which induces retention of body fluids and elicits the stress response. Thoughts for Reflection 7.3, Some Tips on Reducing Sodium in Your Diet, (page 155), provides some ideas for reducing sodium in your diet.

6. *Water* This extremely important constituent of the diet is most often forgotten. We take water for granted most of the time. In the absence of water, life will perish. Water, after oxygen, is the second-most important substance

Table 7.1 IMPORTANT SOURCES OF SOME VITAMINS

Vitamin	Sources
A (retinol)	Eggs, whole milk, fish, green leafy vegetables such as spinach, cabbage, broccoli; colored vegetables such as carrots and pumpkin; fruits such as papaya and mango
B_1 (thiamine)	Dried yeast, unmilled cereals, pork, liver, lentils, nuts, and oilseeds
B_2 (riboflavin)	Liver, meat, milk, yogurt, eggs, cereals, and vegetables
Niacin	Grain products (whole grain, enriched cereals, and bread), milk, poultry, fish, beef, peanut butter, and legumes
B_6 (pyridoxine)	Chicken, fish, kidney, liver, pork, eggs, unmilled rice, soybeans, oats, whole-wheat products, peanuts, and walnuts
Folic acid	Liver, yeast, leafy vegetables, legumes, fortified grain products (bread, cereal, pasta, rice), and some fruits
B_{12}	Meat, eggs, milk, fish, and poultry
C (ascorbic acid)	Green and red peppers, collard greens, broccoli, spinach, tomatoes, potatoes, strawberries, oranges, and other citrus fruits
D	Exposure to sunlight; fortified milk, breakfast cereals, fortified margarine, eggs, salmon, and sardines
E	Vegetable oils (soybean, corn, cottonseed, safflower), raw spinach, almonds, wheat germ, and peanut butter
K	Green leafy vegetables, milk, meats, eggs, cereals, fruits, and vegetables

THOUGHTS FOR
REFLECTION 7.3

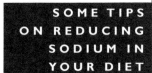

SOME TIPS
ON REDUCING
SODIUM IN
YOUR DIET

At the Store

- Read labels for information on the sodium content.

- Try fresh or plain frozen vegetables and meats instead of those that are canned or prepared with salt.

- Look for low- or reduced-sodium or "no-salt-added" versions of foods.

In the Kitchen

- Cook plain rice, pasta, and hot cereals using less salt than the package calls for (try 1/8 teaspoon of salt for two servings). Instant rice, pasta, and cereals may contain salt added by the processor.

- Adjust your recipes, gradually cutting down on the amount of salt. If some of the ingredients already contain salt, such as canned soup or vegetables, you may not need to add more salt.

- Use herbs and spices as seasonings for vegetables and meats instead of salt.

At the Table

- Taste your food before you salt it. Does it really need more salt? Try one shake instead of two. Gradually cut down on the amount of salt you use. Your taste will adjust to less salt. The greatest sources of sodium in the American diet are processed foods (including restaurant foods).

Note: From Food facts for older adults: Information on how to use the dietary guidelines (pp. 8–9) by Human Nutrition Information Service, U.S. Department of Agriculture and National Institute on Aging, National Institutes of Health, 1993, Hyattsville, MD: U.S. Department of Agriculture.

required for human health. Water helps transport all nutrients, removes waste products, and regulates body temperature. Water is a universal solvent and transport medium, and as a result, it is the basis of all biological processes in the human body. The transport of nutrients can only take place through a solvent, and as such, water acts as the main transport medium of nutrients. Water also helps dilute harmful substances that accumulate in the body and aids in excretion of these substances. Water attends to heat regulation in our bodies. It is of vital importance that body temperature stays at a constant level. That is why we have to drink more water when we have a fever. Water takes up heat and transports it out of the body through perspiration. We can survive without food for about 30 to 40 days, but we can only survive a few days without water.

To combat stress effectively, the body needs an adequate supply of water. Water suppresses the appetite and helps the body metabolize stored fat. The kidneys cannot function properly without enough water. When they do not work properly, some of their load is shifted to the liver. One of the liver's primary functions is to metabolize stored fat into usable energy for the body. If the liver has to do some of the kidney's work, it cannot perform this primary function. As a consequence, fat is deposited. Therefore, drinking water is also helpful in regulating one's body fat.

It is recommended that we drink eight to ten 8-ounce glasses of water every day. This means drinking water when one is not thirsty. If we consume water only when we are thirsty, we have not been drinking a sufficient amount of water. When the human body has less water, the amount of saliva in the mouth tends to decrease. As a result the mouth becomes dry, and this dryness is interpreted as thirst. When we are thirsty, we should not replace water with other beverages, such as soft drinks and so on. We already have seen that beverages such as cola, tea, coffee, and the like contain caffeine and preservatives that do more harm than good (See Box 7.1, Caffeine: What It Is and How Much Is Found in Popular Drinks, page 157). Alcoholic beverages are harmful as they depress the central nervous system, have addictive properties, and are injurious to various parts of the body, such as the liver.

The water we drink should be safe and free from bacteria, viruses, parasitic protozoa, parasitic worms, pesticides, and other chemicals. Some places have hard water. Hard water causes problems in domestic situations such as soap use, as soap is not able to mix with hard water; and hard water can interfere with industrial processes, can plug water pipes, and so on. However, hard water has not been shown to have any adverse health effects.

Water is the only substance in the diet that, for the most part, does no harm to the body in large quantities and has only beneficial results.

avoiding alcohol, smoking, and drug abuse

The issues of alcohol, smoking, and drug abuse are extensive and complex in nature. However, we would like to briefly discuss some points regarding these issues, because many people attempt to find solutions to their stress problems by using, misusing, and abusing chemical substances.

BOX 7·1

Caffeine: What It Is and How Much Is Found in Popular Drinks

Chemically, caffeine is an alkaloid. There are numerous alkaloid compounds. Among them are the methylxanthines, which include three well-known compounds: theophylline (found in tea), theobromine (found in cocoa bean), and caffeine. Caffeine is primarily found in coffee, tea, cola nuts, maté, and guarana and is added to most soft drinks. The primary pharmacological effects of caffeine are as stimulants of the central nervous system, cardiac muscle, and respiratory system. Caffeine also delays fatigue. Pharmacologically, it is labeled as a sympathomimetic agent. When consumed it triggers a response similar to stress.

Most soft drinks today contain caffeine. Below is the caffeine content in milligrams of some popular products:

Product	Caffeine Content (mg)	Size (oz)
Amp	71	8
BuzzWater	200	16.9
Coca-Cola Classic	35	12
Coffee (brewed)	95	8
Coffee (decaf)	2	8
Dr. Pepper	41	12
Full Throttle	144	16
Jolt Cola	72	12
Mello Yellow	53	12
Monster	160	16
Mountain Dew	54	12
Pepsi-Cola	38	12
RC Cola	45.2	12
Red Bull	76	8.3
Rockstar	160	16
SoBe Essential Energy	48	8
SoBe Green Tea	14	8
Shasta Cola	44.4	12
Starbucks Bottled Frappucino	115	9.5
Starbucks Tall Caffe Mocha	95	12
Tea (black, brewed)	47	8
Tea (green)	30	8
Vamp	240	16
Vitamin Energy	150	16
ZipFizz Energy Drink Mix	100	16

Drinking alcoholic beverages is associated with a number of health problems. Alcoholic beverages supply calories to the body but fail to provide any nutrients. These "empty calories" often lead to malnourishment and decreased capabilities in combating daily stresses. Excessive alcohol use has also been associated as a risk factor with cirrhosis of the liver, inflammation of the pancreas, damage to the brain and heart, and increased risk for a variety of cancers. Alcohol is a central nervous system depressant and therefore decreases reaction time, hampers judgment, and impairs sensory responses. As we have seen in Chapters 1 and 2, perception Perception of a stressor is central to the effective management of stress. When this perception is distorted by use of alcohol, recuperation from stress is considerably lowered. Also, there are costs associated with alcohol that can lead to stress. These costs include the direct cost of purchasing alcohol, the possibility of getting tickets or other kinds of fines while under the influence, making poor decisions, and spending money that one would normally not spend. Further, college students who indulge in episodic high drinking called "binge drinking" not only distort their judgment drastically but also increase chances of an accident and even death.

Binge drinking is defined as a pattern of drinking alcohol that brings blood alcohol concentration (BAC) to 0.08 gram percent and above. For the typical adult, this pattern corresponds to consuming five or more drinks (male), or four or more drinks (female), in about 2 hours (National Institute of Alcohol Abuse and Alcoholism, 2004). A drink is a half ounce of alcohol, or one 12-ounce beer, one 5-ounce glass of wine, or 1.5-ounce shot of distilled spirits. This pattern of consumption is common among college students in the United States. Many students use this pattern of drinking to relieve stress.

Surveys done in 1993, 1997, 1999, 2001, and 2005 for college alcohol consumption trends asked about the occurrence of binge drinking in the past two weeks prior to completion of the questionnaire (Nelson, Xuan, Lee, Weitzman, & Wechsler, 2009; Wechsler, Lee, Kuo, & Lee, 2000). The outcome of these surveys showed that the proportion of binge drinkers remained similar in all subgroups and in all types of colleges. Binge drinkers tend to be white males, belonging to a fraternity or a sorority, who had a history of binge drinking in high school. Another study conducted among a nationally representative sample of students across 140 campuses found similar results (Wechsler, Dowdall, Davenport, & Castillo, 1995). The importance of engaging in binge drinking was inextricably linked to the typical aspects of American college life such as parties, athletics, and interactions with friends. Binge drinking continues to be a problem, and prevention efforts in the form of effective interventions are the need of the hour.

Many people smoke because they think that they will get relief from stress. However, this is not true. Tobacco smoke contains nicotine, which is a pseudostressor, as we have already seen in **Worksheet 7.1** (page 163). When the body gets habituated to smoking, it requires more nicotine to get the release of normal chemicals, which may falsely give a smoker the feeling of stress relief. This stress is in fact self-inflicted and can be completely avoided. Tobacco smoke has also been associated with a number of health problems including emphysema, bronchitis, lung cancer, and so on. For a pregnant woman, smoking can lead to low birth weight in her child. If one is a smoker, he or she needs to

THOUGHTS FOR
REFLECTION 7.4

**DIETARY GOALS
TO THINK
ABOUT**

■ To avoid becoming overweight, *consume only as much energy (calories) as is expended*; if overweight, decrease energy intake and increase energy expenditure.

■ The consumption of complex carbohydrates and "naturally occurring" sugars should be about *45 to 65 percent of energy* intake. For a 2,000 calorie diet, 50 percent of energy as carbs would be 1,000 calories/4 cal/g carb = 250 g carb.

■ Reduce the consumption of refined and processed sugars.

■ Total fat should be *20 to 35 percent of the total calories*. Reduce saturated fat consumption to account for no more than 10 percent of total energy intake. Polyunsaturated fats should account for no more than *10 percent of energy intake*; monounsaturated fats should make up the remainder (10 to 15 percent) of total calories.

■ Reduce cholesterol consumption.

■ Limit the intake of sodium.

■ Consume potassium-rich foods, such as fruits and vegetables.

seriously consider quitting. The decision for quitting needs to come from within, then an effective plan can be undertaken.

Most illegal drugs also act on the central nervous system. Some commonly abused and misused drugs are cocaine, marijuana, methamphetamine, heroin, LSD, and so on. These drugs can depress or stimulate the central nervous system or alter and distort sensory responses. In all cases, the net result is poor perception and decreased coping capabilities. Drug abuse also leads to psychological and/or physical dependence. Let's ask ourselves,

❍ Am I resorting to alcohol use, smoking, or drug use to find answers to my problems?

❍ Is this the correct decision?

❍ How else can I solve my problems?

If alcohol or drug abuse is a problem, seek professional help at the earliest possible time. Consider contacting a professional counselor, family physician, or a support organization such as Alcoholics Anonymous (AA). The local address of Alcoholics Anonymous can be found in the telephone book or online.

balanced diet plan for stress reduction and healthful living

The discussion in this chapter has been designed to help you understand the value and importance of maintaining a balanced diet, developing appropriate eating habits, and avoiding negative stress-coping practices such as alcohol and drug abuse. Thoughts for Reflection 7.4, Dietary Goals to Think About, above, will help you ponder some dietary goals that you need to implement in daily life. Now, sharpen your skills in developing and maintaining a diet plan with the help ▶ of **Worksheet 7.2** (page 168).

summary points

○ Sleeping 7 to 8 hours daily, eating breakfast daily, consuming only planned snacks between meals, being at or near prescribed BMI, never smoking, moderate or no use of alcohol, and regular physical activity are some practices associated with good health.

○ A healthy balanced diet when taken at regular times reduces stress and improves stress-coping capabilities.

○ Maintaining weight based upon the ideal range for height is important for healthy living and stress reduction.

○ Coffee, tea, and colas have caffeine, which is a pseudostressor, or a sympathomimetic agent; that is, it produces a stresslike response in the body.

○ Nicotine, which is found in tobacco, is also a sympathomimetic agent and produces stress.

○ Alcohol and illegal drugs do not relieve stress but can only add more stress.

○ Regulating salt and sugar intake in the diet is essential for managing stress.

○ The American Heart Association recommends no more than 2,300 mg of sodium in the diet per day.

○ We need to observe moderation in consuming carbohydrates and proteins in our diet and make healthy choices.

○ Animal fats should be used sparingly.

○ Vitamins and minerals can be taken in recommended and optimum quantities in food sources.

○ Water in the diet is the only constituent that should be taken in large amounts. It is recommended that we drink at least eight to ten 8-ounce glasses of water daily.

important terms defined

binge drinking: Pattern of drinking alcohol that brings blood alcohol concentration (BAC) to 0.08 gram percent and above. For the typical adult this pattern corresponds to consuming five or more drinks (male), or four or more drinks (female), in about 2 hours. A drink refers to a half ounce of alcohol, or one 12-ounce beer, one 5-ounce glass of wine, or 1.5-ounce shot of distilled spirits.

body mass index (BMI): An indicator that is calculated by dividing measured body weight in kilograms by the square of height in meters. The National Institutes of Health (NIH) define normal BMI as 18.5–24.9 (kg/m^2). Overweight is defined as BMI = 25–29.9 (kg/m^2). Class I obesity is 30–34.9 (kg/m^2); Class II obesity is 35–39.9 (kg/m^2); class III (extreme) obesity is > 40 (kg/m^2).

carbohydrate: An organic compound constituted by varying combinations of carbon, hydrogen, and oxygen. Carbohydrates are needed by the body primarily for energy and storage.

cholesterol: A major organic chemical constituent of cell membranes. Synthesized in the body, it is not an essential dietary nutrient. Diets that contain large amounts of cholesterol inhibit synthesis of cholesterol by the body but result in increased cholesterol levels. The average American diet contains more than 450 mg per day of cholesterol, but less than 300 mg is recommended. *See also* **fats**.

electrolytes: Sodium, potassium, and chloride constitute the electrolytes in the body. A healthy balance is needed in these three important chemicals. Conditions such as diarrhea, exercise, less water intake, stress, and some metabolic disorders can alter their balance. These are essential chemicals required by the body for maintaining metabolic balance.

fats: An organic compound formed by fatty acids. Fat is the most concentrated form of energy. Dietary fat also provides the essential fatty acid linoleic acid, which is not synthesized by the body. *See also* **cholesterol**.

mineral: An inorganic element required by the body, typically in a small amount. Examples include calcium, phosphorus, iron, and magnesium.

protein: An organic compound formed by amino acids. The body requires protein for growth and maintenance of body structure and function. Dietary proteins also supply the nine essential amino acids that are not synthesized by the body.

sympathomimetic agent: A chemical, such as caffeine, that resembles the actions of the adrenaline hormone produced by the sympathetic nervous system. These agents stimulate the cardiac muscle, central nervous system, and respiratory system.

vitamin: A member of a heterogeneous group of organic compounds that the body requires for a variety of essential metabolic functions. A vitamin is classified as fat-soluble or water-soluble.

websites to explore

ACADEMY OF NUTRITION AND DIETETICS

www.eatright.org

This website presents useful information from the professional association of dietitians in the United States.

- Visit this website and find out the requirements for becoming a dietitian. Also read the daily healthy tips provided.

CANADA'S FOOD GUIDE

www.healthcanada.gc.ca/foodguide

This website presents the Canadian government's recommendations regarding food.

- Visit this website and compare the USDA MyPlate with Canada's guidelines. Do you notice any similarities? Did you find any differences? Discuss.

CENTER FOR NUTRITION POLICY AND PROMOTION

www.usda.gov/cnpp/

This official U.S. government website provides information about Dietary Guidelines, MyPlate, and the latest reports on healthy nutrition and eating.

▦ Using MyPlate, locate some sample menus. Is your daily diet and exercise routine in-line with the MyPlate recommendations?

DIETARY GUIDELINES FOR AMERICANS, 2010

www.cnpp.usda.gov/DietaryGuidelines.htm

The U.S. Department of Health and Human Services (USDHHS) and U.S. Department of Agriculture (USDA) publish a set of dietary guidelines every five years and this website documents these guidelines. The guidelines provide sound advice for all people over the age of two years.

▦ Visit the website and see what you can do to enrich your diet.

HOLISTIC ONLINE CENTER

www.holistic-online.com/stress

This website underscores a holistic approach to health and stress management. It also discusses nutrition guidelines from a holistic perspective.

▦ Read the guidelines on this website and compare them with the recommendations presented in this book. Do you notice any commonalities and differences? Discuss.

HOW TO KEEP A FOOD JOURNAL

www.ehow.com/how_4723_keep-food-journal.html

This website explains how to record your eating habits and how to interpret your journal. It also provides information about how to eat out, eat on a plane, assess yourself before making a weight loss plan, choose a diet or weight loss plan, and help your family lose weight.

▦ Visit the website, navigate the links, and then keep a food journal for five days.

NUTRITION TODAY

www.nutritiontodayonline.com/

This is the website of the popular magazine Nutrition Today, which publishes articles by leading nutritionists and scientists who endorse scientifically sound food, diet, and nutritional practices.

▦ Navigate this website and review some abstracts that relate to stress and nutrition. These are available free, but in order to see the full text, you may have to pay a price.

Enhancing Awareness About Diet and Eating

Think about the following items and respond to them to obtain feedback regarding your dietary habits and patterns:

1. Height _____

2. Weight _____

3. According to the BMI chart on page 167, is my weight within the healthy range? _____

4. When was the last time I recorded my weight? _____

5. How often do I record my weight?

   _____ Daily

   _____ Weekly

   _____ Every other week

   _____ Monthly

   _____ Every other month

   _____ Quarterly

   _____ Yearly

   _____ Whenever I feel like it

   _____ Sometimes, irregularly

   _____ Never

6. Do I eat breakfast?

   _____ Regularly every day

   _____ Occasionally

   _____ Never

7. Do I eat between meals?

   _____ Always

   _____ Occasionally

   _____ Never

8. Do I drink coffee, tea, or colas?

   _____ Every day   What type? _____

   _____ Occasionally   How much? _____

   _____ Never

(continued)

Enhancing Awareness About Diet and Eating *(cont'd)*

9. Do I use tobacco products?

   _____ Every day   What type? _____

   _____ Occasionally   How much? _____

   _____ Never

10. Do I drink alcoholic beverages?

   _____ Every day   What type? _____

   _____ Occasionally   How much? _____

   _____ Never

11. Do I take any illegal drugs?

   _____ Yes   What type? _____

   _____ No   How much? _____

12. Do I eat the following food items at least once per day? (Put a check mark next to each one that applies.)

   _____ Canned foods

   _____ Processed cheese

   _____ Seasonings

   _____ Sausage/ham/bacon/hamburgers/steaks

   _____ Chips (potato/corn/tortilla)

   _____ Table salt

   _____ Pizza

   _____ Fast food

13. How often do I eat chocolate?

   _____ Never

   _____ Rarely

   _____ Sometimes

   _____ Often

   _____ Daily

Enhancing Awareness About Diet and Eating (cont'd)

14. What is my level of sugar consumption (namely, carbonated beverages and candy)?

_____ Excessive

_____ Moderate

_____ Adequate

_____ Less than normal

FEEDBACK ON WORKSHEET 7.1

Items 1–3 Ideal weight can be determined by studying the body mass index (BMI) chart shown in Figure 7.2 (page 167). Based on height you can determine your healthy weight range, which gives you a BMI of 18.5 to 25.

Items 4–5 You should record your weight regularly. A written record provides a chronologic baseline to compare and make changes as necessary. However, you should not be fanatical about recording weights too often because weight changes are slow to occur. See Figure 7.2 on page 167 to determine whether your current weight is healthy.

Item 6 Research indicates that hypoglycemia, or low blood sugar, may predispose an individual to stress. Although fairly uncommon, symptoms of hypoglycemia may include anxiety, headache, dizziness, trembling, and increased cardiac activity (Girdano, Everly, & Dusek, 2012). The best way to avoid stress associated with hypoglycemia, for a normal person, is to eat a balanced breakfast every day (benefits include intake of essential nutrients, less overeating during the day, better concentration).

Item 7 Eating continuously between meals may unduly activate the digestive system, leading to a release of various chemicals and by-products that may add to stress. This self-induced stress can be controlled by planning to consume food more appropriately. However, research has shown that small meals and healthy snacks can positively influence body weight, blood cholesterol levels, overall nutrition quality, and diet.

Item 8 Coffee, tea, and colas have *caffeine*, which is identified as a **sympathomimetic agent**, or pseudostressor. When consumed, sympathomimetic agents trigger a stress response in the body. An 8-ounce cup of coffee (*Coffea arabica*) contains about 95 milligrams (mg) of caffeine; tea (*Camelia sinensis*) contains 47 mg/cup. Various cola beverages contain 30–60 mg/12 oz, and a bar of chocolate (1 oz) contains about 20 mg of caffeine (Girdano, Everly, & Dusek, 2012).

Item 9 Nicotine found in tobacco is also a sympathomimetic agent and produces a stress response in the body. Tobacco smoke contains various other harmful products, such as tar and carbon monoxide, that can lead to bronchitis, lung cancer, and other diseases.

Item 10 Although it may appear to reduce stress, alcohol is a central nervous system inhibitor. Stress is known to be tied to alcohol addiction (Schlaadt, 1992). There are approximately 10 to 13 million alcoholics in the United States and more than 7 million alcohol abusers. Alcohol abuse is at the root of impaired job performance, child abuse, spouse abuse, accidental injuries, and medical disorders (*Seventh Special Report*, 1990). Further, large numbers of college students indulge in binge drinking, which is very harmful (Hart, Ksir, & Ray, 2010).

(continued)

Item 11 Illegal drugs may be grouped into five categories: *stimulants*, such as cocaine; *marijuana* and its derivatives; *depressants*, such as the opiates; *psychedelics*; *deliriants*; and *designer drugs* (Hart, Ksir & Ray, 2010). These drugs do not relieve stress. In fact, they add to the stress response in the long run. Adopting these negative mechanisms for temporary relief of stress can be extremely hazardous and ruin our physical, mental, and social well-being.

Item 12 Fast foods and other products mentioned in the list are often rich in *sodium* content. Sodium is a mineral responsible for regulating water balance in the body. The United States Recommended Dietary Allowances suggest no more than 2,300 milligrams of sodium per day. If the products you have checked are high in sodium, it is important to restrict their usage. A nutritious diet provides the necessary sodium, and excessive sodium may contribute to an increase in blood pressure and stress (Greenberg, 2010).

Item 13 Chocolate contains *caffeine* and *sugar*. Caffeine, as explained earlier, is a sympathomimetic agent. It induces a response in the body that is akin to the stress response. Excess sugar provides the body with unused energy, and this usually leads to the accumulation of harmful by-products. Both these products therefore add to our stress and need to be avoided. Evidence now indicates that a small to moderate intake of dark chocolate has heart-health benefits.

Item 14 Excessive sugar, as previously explained, leaves excess unused energy in the body. This stored energy does not relieve stress, but in fact adds to stress levels. Moreover, consuming large quantities of sugar over a long period may contribute directly or indirectly to weight gain and various diseases, such as diabetes mellitus. Therefore, it is best to regulate the intake of sugar in our diets.

Increased stress acts as a deviation from homeostasis (balance) in the systems of the body. Elevated blood pressure and increased levels of stress hormones (that is, glucocorticoids) are a sign of stress. Increased body weight, body fat, and insufficient essential nutrient intake, overeating, and undereating all cause stress in the body leading to chronic diseases (that is, deviations from homeostasis). Too much fast food, sugar, and fats creates an imbalance of nutrients. Choosing appropriate foods will counter the stressors built up in the body by inappropriate foods.

BODY MASS INDEX

The **body mass index** (BMI) is now the accepted standard to assess healthy body weight. The USDA (2005) offers the following advice:

> *Choose a lifestyle that combines sensible eating with regular physical activity. To be at their best, adults need to avoid gaining weight, and many need to lose weight. Being overweight or obese increases your risk for high blood pressure, high blood cholesterol, heart disease, stroke, diabetes, certain types of cancer, arthritis, and breathing problems. A healthy weight is key to a long, healthy life… .*
>
> *Keep track of your weight and your waist measurement, and take action if either of them increases. If your BMI is greater than 25, or even if it is in the "healthy" range, at least try to avoid further weight gain. If your waist measurement increases, you are probably gaining fat. If so, take steps to eat fewer calories and become more active (see Dietary Guidelines for Americans).*

HOW TO EVALUATE YOUR WEIGHT (ADULTS):

1. Weigh yourself and measure your height. Find your BMI category using the chart on the following page. The higher your BMI category, the greater the risk for health problems.

2. Measure around your waist, just above your hip bones, while standing. Health risks increase as waist measurement increases, particularly if waist is greater than 35 inches for women or 40 inches for men. Excess abdominal fat may place you at greater risk of health problems, even if your BMI is about right.

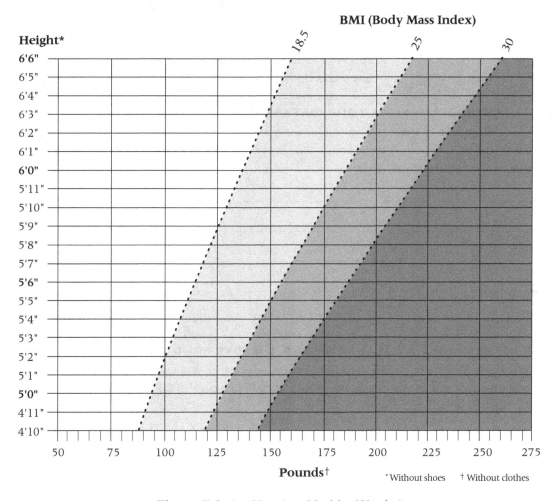

Figure 7.2 Are You At a Healthy Weight?

BMI measures weight in relation to height. The BMI ranges shown above are for adults. They are not exact ranges of healthy and unhealthy weights. However, they show that health risk increases at higher levels of overweight and obesity. Even within the healthy BMI range, weight gains can carry health risks for adults.

Directions: Find your weight on the bottom of the graph. Go straight up from that point until you come to the line that matches your height. Then, look to find your weight group.

Healthy Weight: BMI from 18.5 up to 25 refers to healthy weight.

Overweight: BMI from 25 up to 30 refers to overweight.

Obese: BMI 30 or higher refers to obesity. Obese persons are also overweight.

Note: Report of the Dietary Guidelines Advisory Committee on the Dietary Guidelines for Americans, 2000, P. 3.

Twelve-Step Balanced Diet Plan for Stress Reduction and Healthful Living

Following are 12 steps that will help you plan your diet better for stress reduction and healthful living. Read each step and in the space provided write your own plan for how you would go about accomplishing that step.

STEP 1. BECOMING AWARE OF YOUR DIETARY HABITS

Analyze your dietary habits. Skipping meals intensifies the stress response. The largest meal of the day needs to be taken earlier in the day. Be sure to find out whether you have three meals a day or not. Do you skip any meals? Which is your largest meal of the day?

_____

_____

_____

_____

_____

STEP 2. ESTABLISHING A BALANCE AMONG THE FIVE FOOD GROUPS

The USDA's MyPlate suggests a balance of five food groups emphasizing grains, vegetables, and fruits, while placing less importance on milk products and meat and beans (Figure 7.1 on page 151). Do you include food items from all five food groups in appropriate quantities?

_____

_____

_____

_____

_____

STEP 3. PLANNING TO LIMIT THE INTAKE OF CAFFEINATED BEVERAGES

We have seen that caffeine is a pseudostressor and causes a stress-like response. Therefore, you should work to reduce your intake of caffeinated beverages. Some people like to stop them all at once, whereas others gradually taper their intake, and then substitute their intake with noncaffeinated beverages. Write down and implement a strategy that suits you.

_____

_____

_____

_____

_____

Twelve-Step Balanced Diet Plan for Stress Reduction and Healthful Living (cont'd)

STEP 4. PLANNING TO INCREASE FRUIT AND VEGETABLE CONSUMPTION

For most of us, if we analyze our dietary behavior, we find that we do not consume enough fruits and vegetables in our diet as recommended by the USDA in MyPlate. Do you eat enough servings of fruits? What about vegetables? Write down a strategy to increase the consumption of fruits and vegetables.

_____

_____

_____

_____

_____

_____

STEP 5. PLANNING TO TAKE TIME TO EAT MEALS

Most college students and working adults are eating on the go. Fast food is very popular in our country. Do you take enough time to sit down and eat your meals? Do you take time to eat breakfast? Lunch? Dinner? Write down and allocate at least 30 to 60 minutes for eating each of these three meals.

_____

_____

_____

_____

_____

_____

STEP 6. PLANNING TO LIMIT THE DAILY INTAKE OF SALT IN YOUR DIET

We have seen that salt leads to retention of body water and may cause an increase in blood pressure. You need to avoid using any table salt and work at curbing your intake of fast food and precooked food unless it is absolutely necessary. Work out a strategy to implement this plan.

_____

_____

_____

_____

_____

(continued)

Twelve-Step Balanced Diet Plan for Stress Reduction and Healthful Living *(cont'd)*

STEP 7. PLANNING TO LIMIT THE DAILY INTAKE OF SUGAR

Excessive sugar intake can paradoxically reduce the blood sugar levels, causing hypoglycemia. This result occurs because temporarily high levels of sugar stimulate the release of insulin, which causes blood sugar levels to fall (Smith, 1993). Therefore, limiting the intake of sugar helps in reducing stress. Work out a strategy to limit your sugar intake.

_____

_____

_____

_____

_____

STEP 8. PLANNING TO STOP SMOKING

We have seen that smoking does not reduce stress. As discussed earlier, nicotine found in tobacco has an addictive effect on the stress response. To begin with, keep a record of the number of cigarettes smoked and seek support from close friends. You then need to work at delaying the urge to smoke as many times as possible during the day. This purpose can be achieved by diverting the mind to do something else at the time of the urge and replacing the smoking habit with other constructive habits (for example, exercising). In this way, you can consistently work at cutting the number of cigarettes you smoke. Finally, you need to decide upon a day, and quit smoking completely. You need to adhere to this commitment religiously. Work out a definitive plan for yourself to quit smoking.

_____

_____

_____

_____

_____

Twelve-Step Balanced Diet Plan for Stress Reduction and Healthful Living (cont'd)

STEP 9. PLANNING TO AVOID OR REDUCE ALCOHOL INTAKE

Moderation in intake of alcohol and alcoholic beverages is vital in order to maintain balance and avoid stress. If you are not now practicing moderation, write out a plan to work at establishing it.

_____

_____

_____

_____

_____

_____

STEP 10. SUPPLEMENTING VITAMINS AND MINERALS IN THE DIET

Establishing a balance in the daily intake of vitamins and minerals in the diet increases resistance to stress. It is best to choose a wide variety of foods to meet one's vitamin and mineral needs in place of supplements (see Table 7.1 on page 155). Write out a plan to ensure that the needed vitamins and minerals are included in your diet.

_____

_____

_____

_____

_____

_____

_____

STEP 11. UTILIZING NATURAL FOOD PRODUCTS

Natural food products, such as yogurt, have been suggested to help improve stress-coping capabilities. One of the components of yogurt, _Lactobacillus acidophilus_, has received attention. These bacteria are harmless and have been claimed to inhibit growth of pathogenic bacteria, boost the immune system, produce essential vitamins, and enhance resistance to stress (Chaitow & Trenev, 1990; Lee, 1988; Schauss, 1990). Plan to increase consumption of natural food products in your diet.

_____

_____

_____

_____

_____

_____

(continued)

Twelve-Step Balanced Diet Plan for Stress Reduction and Healthful Living *(cont'd)*

STEP 12. MAINTAINING WEIGHT THROUGH REGULAR MONITORING AND CONTROL

To reduce stress in your life, maintaining weight by weekly or bimonthly monitoring and working out an effective diet and exercise plan are vital. What is your plan?

_____

_____

_____

_____

_____

_____

references and further readings

Belloc, N. B., & Breslow, L. (1972). Relationship of physical health status and health practices. *Preventive Medicine*, 1, 409–421.

Chaitow, L., & Trenev, N. (1990). *Probiotics: The revolutionary "friendly bacteria" way to vital health and well being.* Northamptonshire: Thorsons.

Cuthbertson, D. P. (1964). Physical injury and its effects on protein metabolism. In H. H. Munro & J. B. Allison (Eds.), *Mammalian protein metabolism* (vol. 2, pp. 374–414). New York: Academic Press.

Flegal, K.M., Carroll, M.D., Kuczmarski, R.J., & Johnson, C.L. (1998). Overweight and obesity in the United States: Prevalence and trends, 1960–1994. *International Journal of Obesity and Related Metabolic Disorders*, 22(1), 39–47.

Flegal, K. M., Carroll, M. D., Kit, B. K., & Ogden, C. L. (2012). Prevalence of obesity and trends in the distribution of body mass index among US adults, 1999-2010. *JAMA*, 307(5), 491–497.

Food and Nutrition Board, Institute of Medicine. *Dietary Reference Intake for Energy, Carbohydrate, Fiber, Fat, Fatty Acids, Cholesterol, Protein, and Amino Acids* (2002). Washington, DC: National Press.

Girdano, D. E., Everly, G. S., Jr., & Dusek, D. E. (2012). *Controlling stress and tension: A holistic approach* (9th ed.). Englewood Cliffs, NJ: Prentice Hall.

Greenberg, J. S. (2010). *Comprehensive stress management* (12th ed.). Boston: McGraw-Hill.

Hart, C. L., Ksir, C., & Ray, O. (2010). *Drugs, society, and human behavior* (14th ed.). Boston: Brown/Mcgraw-Hill.

Lee, W. H. (1988). *The friendly bacteria: How lactobacilli and bifidobacteria can transform your health.* New Canaan, CT: Keats.

National Institute of Alcohol Abuse and Alcoholism. (2004, Winter). Binge drinking defined. National Institute of Alcohol Abuse and Alcoholism Newsletter, 3, 3.

Nelson, T. F., Xuan, Z., Lee, H., Weitzman, E. R., & Wechsler, H. (2009). Persistence of heavy drinking and ensuing consequences at heavy drinking colleges. *Journal of Studies on Alcohol and Drugs*, 70(5), 726–734.

Schauss, A. G. (1990). Lactobacillus acidophilus: Method of action, clinical application and toxicity data. *Journal of Advancement in Medicine*, 3, 163–178.

Schlaadt, R. G. (1992). *Alcohol use and abuse.* Guilford, CT: Dushkin.

Smith, J. C. (1993). *Understanding stress and coping.* New York: Macmillan.

U.S. Department of Agriculture. (2012). Dietary guidelines for Americans, 2010. Retrieved from http://www.cnpp.usda.gov/DietaryGuidelines.htm.

U.S. Department of Health and Human Services. (2005). Dietary Guidelines for Americans, 2005. Retrieved November 15, 2005, from http://www.healthierus.gov/dietaryguidelines/. Washington, DC: U.S. Public Health Service.

U.S. Department of Health and Human Services, Public Health Service, Alcohol, Drug Abuse, and Mental Health Administration, National Institute on Alcohol Abuse and Alcoholism. (1990, January). Seventh Special Report to the U.S. Congress on Alcohol and Health.

Wechsler, H., Dowdall, G.W., Davenport, A., & Castillo, S.(1995). Correlates of college student binge drinking. *American Journal of Public Health*, 85(7), 921–926.

Wechsler, H., Lee, J. E., Kuo, M., & Lee, H. (2000). College binge drinking in the 1990's: A continuing problem. *Journal of American College Health*, 48(5), 199.

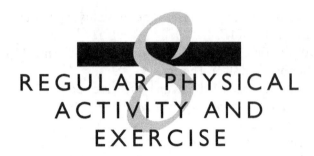

REGULAR PHYSICAL ACTIVITY AND EXERCISE

STRESS
MANAGEMENT
PRINCIPLE

Start a physical activity program, and keep exercising consistently.

importance of physical activity and exercise

Physical activity and **exercise** not only are good for physical health but also enhance mental health. Improvement in both these dimensions positively contributes toward coping with stress effectively. Physical activity and exercise, when performed regularly, promote health by:

○ Providing higher energy levels

○ Improving bodily resistance to disease

○ Improving cardiovascular and respiratory fitness

○ Enhancing self-esteem and confidence

○ Regulating sleep patterns

○ Improving the ability to concentrate

○ Increasing strength and stamina

○ Bringing about an overall positive and healthy outlook to life

Various studies have supported the usefulness of regular physical activity and exercise (Allen & Morelli, 2011; Nam, 2011; Soares-Miranda et al., 2011). Paffenberger and colleagues (1993) demonstrated that regular exercise during leisure time can protect people against premature death from any cause, particularly coronary heart disease. The exact mechanism by which physical activity and exercise operate to reduce the incidence of coronary heart disease is debatable. A number of theories have been presented. Some researchers theorize that it is due to modification of feelings such as anger (Czajkowski et al., 1990); some attribute it to physiological

BOX 8·1

Physical Activity: Benefits and Recommendations from the Surgeon General's Report (2004)

Regular physical activity is helpful in preventing and controlling morbidity and premature mortality associated with a number of chronic diseases. The chief benefits of regular physical activity include:

- Prevention and control of coronary heart disease (CHD), stroke, non-insulin-dependent diabetes mellitus, hypertension (high blood pressure), osteoporosis, colon cancer, depression, anxiety, and obesity

- Improved heart, lung, and circulatory system functioning

- Better balance of blood lipids as a result of increasing "good cholesterol," or high-density lipoproteins (HDL), and lowering "bad cholesterol," or low-density lipoproteins (LDL)

- Improved quality of life

- Enhanced functional independence

- Mental well-being

- Counterbalancing of adverse effects due to stress

- Improved self-esteem

- Maintenance of appropriate body weight

- Slowing down the adverse effects of aging such as memory loss

- Overall improved life expectancy

Current recommendations from the Surgeon General's Report include the following:

- A goal of 60 minutes per day of moderate-intensity activities on most days of the week

- Utilization of recreational activities, such as jogging, bicycling, and swimming, in daily life

- Inclusion of lifestyle activities, such as climbing stairs, mowing the lawn, or walking to and from work, in everyday routine

reasons such as increased blood flow to the brain or release of endorphins (Smith, 1993); and, finally, others believe it is due to diversion of attention from daily hassles and an accompanying relief in stress (Bahrke & Morgan, 1978). Whatever the exact mechanism is, there is a great deal of positive evidence in support of regular physical activity and exercise.

In 1996, the U.S. Department of Health and Human Services released the first Surgeon General's Report to address physical activity and health. The primary message of this report was that Americans can substantially improve their health and quality of life by incorporating moderate amounts of physical activity in their lives. With regard to stress-related disorders, the report pointed out that physical activity appeared to relieve symptoms of depression and anxiety and improve mood. In the wake of these recommendations, it makes a lot of sense to include regular exercise and physical activity in one's lifestyle to reduce stress and manage it better. See Box 8.1, Physical Activity: Benefits and Recommendations from the Surgeon General's Report (2004), above.

The American College of Sports Medicine (ACSM) has developed a set of guidelines for healthy aerobic activity for adults (Garber et al., 2011):

- Engage in moderate-intensity cardiorespiratory exercise training for ≥30 minutes per day on ≥5 days per week for a total of ≥150 minutes per week.

- Engage in vigorous-intensity cardiorespiratory exercise training for ≥20 minutes per day on ≥3 days per week (≥75 minutes per week), or a combination of moderate- and vigorous-intensity exercise to achieve a total energy expenditure of ≥500–1000 MET (Metabolic Equivalent of Task) per week.

- Perform resistance exercises for each of the major muscle groups, and neuromotor exercise involving balance, agility, and coordination 2–3 days per week.

- Must complete a series of flexibility exercises for each of the major muscle-tendon groups (a total of 60 seconds per exercise) on ≥2 days per week.

healthy lifestyle

If we are not already engaged in regular physical activity, we have to consider changing our lifestyle. When faced with decisions about change, we need to become more aware of the importance of managing ourselves. We may have limited control over any change affecting our personal lives, family, or work setting, but we can always exercise some control of our lifestyle. Managing ourselves when faced with change involves mobilizing assets and creating strategies for moving through the process. Feeling that we are powerless and helpless when facing a decision that requires change is common. Often we focus on what we cannot control and become victims. When confronted with a decision to change, the goal is not to move others to change. It is more appropriate for us to accept change and plan to move toward our new goals (Krampf & Romas, 2002).

types of exercise

A number of classifications are available to describe types of exercise. From a *biological* point of view, depending upon the oxygen utilization by the body, exercise can be classified into two types:

1. **Aerobic exercise** (*aerobic* meaning "with oxygen") can be defined as exercise that does not require greater oxygen than can be taken in by the body. Examples of aerobic activities include running, walking briskly, jogging, bicycling, swimming, and rope jumping.

2. **Anaerobic exercise** (*anaerobic* meaning "without oxygen") can be defined as exercise in which the body goes all out and the muscles rely heavily on production of energy without adequate oxygen. Examples of anaerobic activity would be sprinting 100 or 200 meters with maximum effort.

This classification is more theoretical in its connotation. According to a *functional* point of view, exercise can be classified into the following types:

1. *Exercise for Circulatory and Respiratory Fitness* The circulatory system consists of the heart, blood, and blood vessels. The blood is an essential carrier of oxygen to all cells of the body. Oxygen is utilized by the cells to produce energy necessary for daily activities. The respiratory system consists of the airways and lungs. The air that we breathe in is taken up by the lungs, and oxygen is supplied to the blood. Therefore, both the circulatory and the respiratory systems are important in supplying oxygen to provide necessary energy to the body. Good oxygenation plays a vital role in managing stress. Examples of activities that improve circulatory and respiratory fitness include brisk walking, jogging, running, and aerobic dancing.

2. *Exercise for Enhancing Muscular Strength and Endurance* Muscular strength is the ability to achieve maximal performance. Muscular endurance is the ability to work continuously for a long period of time. Examples of activities that improve muscular strength and endurance include push-ups, sit-ups, chin-ups, and weight training.

3. *Exercise for Improving Body Flexibility* Flexibility is the ability of the body to perform various motions around the joints. Some activities that promote flexibility are stretching, shoulder reach, trunk flexion, trunk extension, and so on.

4. *Exercise for Reducing Body Fat* Fat is normally deposited around the waist for men and on the thighs for women. Fat deposition also leads to atherosclerotic changes in arteries (narrowing with fatty deposition) and greater risk for coronary heart disease. Generally, exercise activities performed for circulatory and respiratory fitness and muscular strength, described previously, also help in burning off fat.

From an **operational** point of view, based upon the method of performance, exercise can be classified as follows:

1. *Interval training* includes exercising in bouts of hard exercise separated by bouts of light exercise.

2. *Continuous training* includes exercising at a constant, rhythmic level of intensity for a long and uninterrupted period.

3. *Circuit training* includes completing a round of exercises known as a circuit. This circuit can be repeated for a desirable length of time and pace.

From an **applied practical** point of view, exercise can be classified as follows:

1. *Competitive* exercise includes performing for the purpose of competition—that is, in order to win an event. Competitive exercise may produce great distress. One way to prevent this type of negative stress is to avoid competitive sports. If participation in competitive sports is inevitable, or one has a desire to do so, then one has to learn and develop appropriate coping skills in order to avoid potential negative consequences from stress. Such strategies include accepting loss, playing for relaxation, and positive thinking.

2. *Semicompetitive* exercise normally begins as a noncompetitive event, but when one gets into the mood, then one starts competing with others. This competition can also produce stress, and therefore, appropriate coping skills are required.

3. *Noncompetitive* exercise is performed purely for one's own health and satisfaction. There is no element of competition of any kind. This kind of exercise does not produce any negative consequences associated with stress. On the other hand, noncompetitive exercise helps in counteracting the negative consequences of stress.

From the perspective of preventing, reducing, controlling, and managing stress, any noncompetitive aerobic exercise performed rhythmically, with regularity, is most beneficial. Examples of some activities that meet these criteria are:

- *Jogging and Running*—Jogging and running are quite popular in the United States and are very simple. They require no special training and can be performed in almost any location and at any time of the day. All one needs is a good pair of running shoes and appropriate clothing. One also needs to have an empty stomach—that is, not having eaten anything for at least 3 to 4 hours. These activities can be performed individually or in groups. They are excellent aerobic and rhythmic activities and excellent for preventing, reducing, and managing stress.

- *Brisk Walking*—For older persons and people not used to exercising, brisk walking can be a very important initiating exercise. A walking technique needs to be natural and rhythmic. Use of correct posture and proper shoes are also important. This most inexpensive form of exercise, performed regularly, can yield rich dividends.

- *Cycling*—Cycling is also an aerobic rhythmic, cardiorespiratory exercise and is quite helpful in preventing, reducing, and managing stress. For this purpose, cycling needs to be performed noncompetitively either outdoors, in a velodrome, or on a stationary bicycle. For adequate results, this activity needs to be done regularly for 30 minutes at least three to four times a week.

- *Swimming*—Swimming has often been called the most complete form of exercise. Swimming improves cardiorespiratory fitness, flexibility, muscular strength, and endurance. A significant advantage of swimming is that because the body is supported by water, risk of harm to joints and muscles is minimal. This activity is an effective means to prevent, reduce, and manage stress.

- *Cross-Country Skiing*—Cross-country skiing also provides cardiorespiratory and muscular benefits. The whole body is utilized when performing this exercise. This activity is also helpful in preventing, reducing, and managing stress. It may appear that this activity can only be performed outdoors in the winter, but this is not so. One can also perform this activity indoors with the help of artificial equipment.

- *Aerobic Dancing*—Aerobic dancing helps the whole body obtain adequate cardiorespiratory fitness, flexibility, and muscular endurance. In this activity, the mind is constantly engaged in achieving rhythmic coordination, and therefore, this focus helps divert attention from stress-producing thoughts.

- *Activities Involving Use of Any Racquet*—Activities such as racquetball, tennis, table tennis, badminton, and squash, if played noncompetitively, are helpful forms of exercise for improving cardiorespiratory fitness, flexibility, muscular strength, and endurance. These activities also relieve one from the potential harmful negative consequences of stress.

Cross training, or participating in a variety of physical activities, is quite helpful because it provides fun, variety, and choice. It releases bodily strain from different parts of the body.

Before you initiate and sustain a physical activity and exercise program, become more aware of your physical activity levels by completing **Worksheet 8.1** on page 183. **Worksheet 8.2** (page 184) will help you to determine target heart rates

PRINCIPLES OF CONDITIONING FOR PHYSICAL ACTIVITY AND EXERCISE

Conditioning the Mind

- Think about the benefits of a physical activity and exercise program.

- Try to visualize what a physical activity and exercise program can do for you.

- You have to find time for physical activity and exercise. You can find sufficient time even if your schedule is extremely busy. Time availability needs to be created in the mind first.

- Think of any friends or family members who can help monitor your physical activity and exercise. Enter into an agreement with them.

- Be prepared to face a little discomfort in the form of aches and pains in the beginning when you initiate a physical activity and exercise program.

Conditioning the Body

- Increase your physical activity and exercise levels *slowly*. You should not initiate vigorous exercise suddenly. It's best to build up exercise levels slowly and gradually.

- You should remember to start a physical activity and exercise program by *warming up* your body for at least 10 minutes. This warm-up should include activities performed at a slower pace.

- After the warming-up phase you can go into the *conditioning* phase. You have to be careful not to overdo this phase. One of the criteria for judging the intensity is to find your *target heart rate* (see **Worksheet 8.2** on page 184) and not exceed this rate for 15 to 30 minutes.

- You always have to remember to *cool down* for 5 to 10 minutes after the intensive conditioning phase so that the heart rate comes back to near normal. Any easy-paced activity will help you cool down after the strenuous conditioning phase.

- Maintaining regularity in physical activity and exercise is vital for achieving maximum benefits.

---

appropriate for you while performing physical activity. Thoughts for Reflection 8.1, Principles of Conditioning for Physical Activity and Exercise, above, will help you become familiar with some principles for conditioning the body.

initiating and sustaining a regular physical activity or exercise program

We have discussed the importance of physical activity. We have also familiarized ourselves with the various principles required for conditioning the body and mind in order to prepare for exercise. Now we need to work toward initiating and sustaining regular physical activity. **Worksheet 8.3** (page 185) has been designed to facilitate achieving this regularity. It is hoped that this worksheet will foster insights into your behavior and help you adopt a physically active lifestyle. Thoughts for Reflection 8.2, Cautions with Physical Activity (page 180), presents some cautions that you need to keep in mind before, during, and after physical activity.

THOUGHTS FOR
REFLECTION 8.2

**CAUTIONS
WITH
PHYSICAL
ACTIVITY**

■ You should not start vigorous physical activity suddenly. You have to make a plan before you implement it.

■ You have to be careful not to overexert. Common signs of overexertion are:

— Frequent headaches

— Breathing difficulties and shortness of breath

— Excessive tiredness and fatigue that last a long time

— Nausea or vomiting after exercise

— Severe pain all over the body, especially in overworked muscles

— Inability to perform daily activities

— Excessive strain of any part of the body

— Irritability

— Lowered mood

— Sleep disturbances

— Increased resting heart rate

— Decline in physical activity performance

■ Be aware of abnormal signs when being physically active. Common abnormal signs are:

— Chest pain

— Dizziness, fainting

— Seizures

— Irregular heart movements felt as palpitations

— Sustained pain in the joints

— Swelling in any part of the body after exercise

■ Drink plenty of water and fluids that have electrolytes to avoid getting dehydrated.

■ Do not exercise when your stomach is full. You should wait at least 2 hours before exercising if you have eaten something.

■ During pregnancy, the expectant mother should consult her physician before following a regular exercise schedule.

■ Wear a comfortable outfit. Do not wear very tight clothes. Your shoes need to be selected carefully and not cause blisters, corns, or sores.

CHAPTER REVIEW

summary points

○ Regular physical activity and exercise promote health by providing higher energy levels, improving resistance to disease, enhancing self-esteem and confidence, increasing strength and stamina, and bringing about an overall positive and healthy outlook to life.

○ Regular physical activity and exercise help prevent, reduce, control, and manage stress.

○ Biologically, exercise can be classified as aerobic and anaerobic.

○ Functionally, exercise can be classified as activities improving cardiorespiratory fitness, activities enhancing muscular strength and endurance, activities improving body flexibility, and activities reducing fat.

○ Operationally, exercise can be classified as interval, continuous, and circuit training.

○ Practically, exercise can be classified as competitive, semicompetitive, and noncompetitive.

○ For physical activity and exercise to produce optimum benefits for cardiorespiratory fitness and for prevention, reduction, and management of stress, the physical activity and exercise levels need to reach target heart rate for at least 15 to 30 minutes.

○ Conditioning the body and mind are prerequisites for initiating and sustaining any physical activity and exercise program.

○ Steps of an ideal physical activity and exercise program include *warm-up* (10 minutes), *conditioning* (maintaining the target heart rate for 15 to 30 minutes), and *cooldown* (10 minutes).

○ Regularity in physical activity and exercise is extremely important in order to obtain maximum benefits.

important terms defined

aerobic exercise: Physical activity that does not require more oxygen than that which can be taken in by the body. Some examples of aerobic exercise include running, walking, jogging, and swimming. *See also* **anaerobic exercise**.

anaerobic exercise: Physical activity that requires the body to go all out, during which the muscles rely heavily on production of energy without adequate oxygen supply. Some examples of these activities include sprinting and lifting weights. *See also* **aerobic exercise**.

exercise: A planned, structured, and repetitive bodily movement done to improve or maintain one or more components of physical fitness. Areas of physical fitness include cardiorespiratory (such as heart and lung functions), muscular (such as power), metabolic (such as glucose tolerance), morphological (such as body composition), and motor (such as agility).

websites to explore

AMERICAN HEART ASSOCIATION

www.americanheart.org

This is the website of the American Heart Association, a nonprofit organization dedicated to preventing and controlling heart diseases.

▪ Under the Getting Healthy link, visit the Physical Activity link. Read about the tips for increasing physical activity in your life at your home and at play. Which tip appeals to you most? How will you go about incorporating exercise in your life?

CENTERS FOR DISEASE CONTROL AND PREVENTION

www.cdc.gov/nccdphp/dnpa/physical/everyone

This website of the Centers for Disease Control and Prevention has links to physical activities for everyone.

■ Review the resources for health professionals. There are several programs listed on that link. Which program did you like and why?

DEPARTMENT OF HEALTH AND HUMAN SERVICES REPORT ON PHYSICAL ACTIVITY

http://aspe.hhs.gov/health/reports/physicalactivity/

This website offers access to a 2002 report on physical activity and health by the U.S. Department of Health and Human Services.

■ Look up the BMI weight chart presented in the report (Figure 8). Where does your weight fall? Are you healthy, overweight, or obese? What will you do to maintain a healthy weight or arrive in a healthy weight range?

HEALTH CANADA—PHYSICAL ACTIVITY

www.phac-aspc.gc.ca/hp-ps/hl-mvs/pa-ap/04paap-eng.php

This website maintained by the government of Canada provides links to several tips for physical activity in different age groups.

■ Visit this website and choose physical activity tips relevant to your situation. What is one tip that you like most in this website? How will you apply it in your life?

WORLD HEALTH ORGANIZATION

www.who.int/dietphysicalactivity/factsheet_recommendations/en/index.html

This is the website of the World Health Organization, the United Nations specialized agency for health, established in 1948 and committed to ensuring the attainment of the highest possible level of health by all people of the world.

■ Visit this website and read about the global recommendations for physical activity. How are these similar and different than ACSM guidelines? What can you do to reduce physical inactivity at the global level?

WORKSHEET 8.1

This worksheet is available online at www.pearsonhighered.com/romas.

Enhancing Self-Awareness About Physical Activity and Exercise Levels

Circle the choice that best describes your behavior pertaining to physical activity.

	Low		Moderate		High
1. Level of physical activity at work	1	2	3	4	5
2. Level of physical activity at leisure	1	2	3	4	5
3. Regularity of physical activity	1	2	3	4	5
4. Number of times per week	0	1–2	3–4	5–6	>6
5. Duration of physical activity	<15 min.		15–30/30–45 min.		>45 min.

6. Describe the type of physical activity you do:

_____

_____

_____

_____

_____

_____

_____

_____

_____

_____

FEEDBACK ON WORKSHEET 8.1

From the point of view of preventing, reducing, controlling, and managing stress, physical activity needs to be rhythmic, aerobic, noncompetitive, and performed for an adequate amount of time. This worksheet should have provided you with insight on your behavior regarding physical activity. If your physical activity levels are low, then you need to increase them. If your physical activity levels are already high, then you need to sustain these efforts and attain regularity.

If the types of physical activity you are performing are not holistic—that is, if they do not contribute much to all the dimensions including cardiorespiratory fitness, flexibility, muscular strength, and endurance—then you need to choose activities that contribute to all the dimensions. Some activities that have been described earlier include jogging/running, brisk walking, cycling, swimming, cross-country skiing, aerobic dancing, and activities involving the use of a racquet. You should remember to include the components of rhythm, aerobics, and regularity in your exercise schedule.

Calculating Appropriate Target Heart-Rate Range

For physical activity to produce optimum benefits for cardiorespiratory fitness and prevention of stress, physical activity levels need to reach the target heart-rate range for at least 15 to 30 minutes. To calculate your target heart-rate range for being physical active:

1. Subtract your age from 220. Call this A.

   220 − Your age = _____ (A)

2. Take your pulse in a resting state for 1 minute. To do so, take your pulse for 10 seconds, and multiply this number by six. It is best to record your pulse before getting up from bed in the morning to get a true resting heart rate. You can feel the radial pulse at the wrist toward the side of the thumb (against the radius bone) or the carotid pulse in the neck to the side of the Adam's apple. Use your index or middle finger to feel the pulse. Call this B.

   B = _____ beats per minute

3. Subtract B from A. Call this C.

   A − B = _____ − _____ = _____ (C)

4. Multiply C by 0.6. Call the result D.

   C _____ × 0.6 = _____ (D)

5. Add B and D to obtain the *lower end* of your target heart-rate range.

   B + D = _____ + _____ = _____

6. Multiply C by 0.8. Call the result E.

   C _____ × 0.8 = _____ (E)

7. Add B and E to obtain the *upper end* of your target heart-rate range.

   B + E = _____ + _____ = _____

FEEDBACK ON WORKSHEET 8.2

This worksheet should have provided you with an appropriate target heart-rate range specific for your age. When being physically active, it is extremely important to adhere to this target heart-rate range and not exceed the upper limit at any time. This target heart-rate range can be monitored while performing the exercise by taking your own pulse. If you are exceeding the target heart-rate range, then you need to slow down. Another rough method of estimating this is the "talk test." According to this method, if you are able to maintain normal conversation while exercising, then you are likely within the target heart-rate range.

You need to remain within the target heart-rate range for 15 to 30 minutes in the conditioning phase of physical activity. Only after regular physical activity and exercise for 6 months to 1 year can this period be exceeded. We recommend that you do not exceed this period unless you want to become a professional athlete.

It is also important to slowly and *not* suddenly achieve the target heart-rate range. That is why it is recommended that you initiate any physical activity with *warming up* and *stretching*. It is equally important to slowly and not suddenly return to the normal heart-rate range after being in the target heart-rate range for 15 to 30 minutes. Therefore, it is recommended that you complete any physical activity with a slow *cooldown*. This caution acquires greater significance as you grow older.

Five Steps Toward Initiation and Sustenance of a Physical Activity or Exercise Program

Following are five steps that will help you initiate and sustain a physical activity or exercise program. Read the text associated with each step. In the space provided, write down your own plan as to how you would go about accomplishing that step.

STEP 1. DETERMINING YOUR PHYSICAL ACTIVITY OR EXERCISE LEVELS

An awareness about your physical activity or exercise levels is the first step toward developing your own plan of improvement. In the space provided, based upon feedback from **Worksheet 8.1** (page 183), rate your physical activity or exercise levels and write down what, how, and how much you need to improve.

_____

_____

_____

_____

_____

STEP 2. CHECKING BEFORE PHYSICAL ACTIVITY OR EXERCISE

Before initiating a physical activity or exercise program, respond to the following questions. If you answer yes or are not sure about any of the following questions, you should consult your physician before beginning a physical activity or exercise program.

■ Is there a history of heart disease in my family?

_____Yes _____ No _____ Not sure

■ Have I ever been diagnosed to have any heart disease?

_____Yes _____ No _____ Not sure

■ Have I ever suffered from chest pains?

_____Yes _____ No _____ Not sure

■ Do I have shortness of breath while climbing up a flight of stairs?

_____Yes _____ No _____ Not sure

(continued)

Five Steps Toward Initiation and Sustenance
of a Physical Activity or Exercise Program (*cont'd*)

■ Have I ever been diagnosed to have diabetes mellitus, had high blood sugar or sugar in urine detected, or had complaints of excessive hunger, thirst, or increased urination?

_____ Yes _____ No

■ Am I a smoker?

_____ Yes _____ No

■ Am I over 35 years of age and have not exercised regularly?

_____ Yes _____ No

■ Have I ever been diagnosed to have high serum cholesterol levels (particularly LDL (low-density lipoproteins), or "bad cholesterol")?

_____ Yes _____ No

■ Am I taking any prescribed medication(s)?

_____ Yes _____ No

■ Do I have any other medical problems or disabilities?

_____ Yes _____ No

STEP 3. STARTING A PHYSICAL ACTIVITY OR EXERCISE PROGRAM

Having decided that you want to initiate a physical activity or exercise program, you have to choose an appropriate place. Exercise or be physically active either early in the morning, when your stomach is empty, or late in the afternoon, before dinner. It is important to remember that physical activity habits need to be changed gradually. You should increase the duration of exercise by 1 to 5 minutes every other session.

A physical activity or exercise program always has three parts: *warm-up, conditioning*, and *cooldown*. You should practice all three stages meticulously. Now is the time to make a plan to start your physical activity or exercise program if you do not already have one.

_____

_____

_____

_____

_____

_____

_____

Five Steps Toward Initiation and Sustenance
of a Physical Activity or Exercise Program *(cont'd)*

STEP 4. BRAVING THE INITIAL "TEETHING" PROBLEMS

You will likely feel pain, discomfort, and tiredness in the initial few days of starting a physical activity or exercise plan. To be prepared for these, write down in the following space all the anticipated problems you are likely to face, and how you are going to manage them. This step will help you adapt to change in your physical activity or exercise plan.

_____

_____

_____

_____

_____

_____

_____

STEP 5. SUSTAINING REGULARITY IN PHYSICAL ACTIVITY OR EXERCISE

Just as the plant in the pot withers away without regular replenishment by water, any good habit, if not incorporated into a regular plan, does not provide us with complete benefits. Now you should make a plan for yourself as to how you would like to sustain your physical activity or exercise program.

_____

_____

_____

_____

_____

_____

_____

references and further readings

ACSM (American College of Sports Medicine). (2001). *Guidelines for physical activity.* Retrieved Oct. 15, 2002 from *http://www.acsm.org.*

Allen, J., & Morelli, V. (2011). Aging and exercise. *Clinics in Geriatric Medicine, 27*(4), 661–671.

Bahrke, M. S., & Morgan, W. P. (1978). Anxiety reduction following exercise and meditation. *Cognitive Therapy and Research, 2,* 323–333.

Czajkowski, S. M., Hindelang, R. D., Dembroski, T. M., Mayerson, S. E., Parks, E. B., & Holland, J. C. (1990). Aerobic fitness, psychological characteristics, and cardiovascular reactivity to stress. *Health Psychology, 9,* 676–692.

Garber, C. E., Blissmer, B., Deschenes, M. R., Franklin, B. A., Lamonte, M. J., Lee, I. M., Nieman, D. C., Swain, D. P., & American College of Sports Medicine. (2011). American College of Sports Medicine position stand. Quantity and quality of exercise for developing and maintaining cardiorespiratory, musculo-skeletal, and neuromotor fitness in apparently healthy adults: guidance for prescribing exercise. *Medicine and Science in Sports and Exercise, 43*(7), 1334–1359.

Girdano, D. E., Everly, G. S., Jr., & Dusek, D. E. (2008). *Controlling stress and tension: A holistic approach* (8th ed.). Englewood Cliffs, NJ: Prentice Hall.

Greenberg, J. S. (2008). *Comprehensive stress management* (10th ed.). Boston: McGraw-Hill.

Krampf, H., & Romas, J. A. (2002). *Profiles of physical activity for healthy lifestyles.* Dubuque, IA: Kendall Hunt.

Nam, G. B. (2011). Exercise, heart and health. *Korean Circulation Journal, 41*(3), 113–121.

Paffenberger, R. S., Jr., Hyde, R. T., Wing, A. L., Lee, I. M., Jung, D. L., & Kampert, J. B. (1993). The association of changes in physical activity level and other life-style characteristics with mortality among men. *New England Journal of Medicine, 328,* 538–545.

Smith, J. C. (1993). *Understanding stress and coping.* New York: Macmillan.

Soares-Miranda, L., Sandercock, G., Vale, S., Silva, P., Moreira, C., Santos, R., & Mota, J. (2011). Benefits of achieving vigorous as well as moderate physical activity recommendations: Evidence from heart rate complexity and cardiac vagal modulation. *Journal of Sports Sciences, 29*(10), 1011-1018.

U.S. Department of Health and Human Services. (2004). *Physical activity and health: A Report of the Surgeon General.* Atlanta, GA: USDHHS, Centers for Disease Control and Prevention, National Center for Chronic Disease Prevention and Health Promotion.

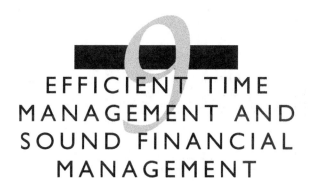

EFFICIENT TIME MANAGEMENT AND SOUND FINANCIAL MANAGEMENT

importance of time management

Time is one of our most precious resources. All of us have the same time available to us, and this time is limited. Our existence on Earth has a limited time frame. We are not even aware how much time is available in our life. Therefore, we need to make the best use of our time. Moreover, the way we use this time determines success in accomplishing our desired goals. In present times, this success is an important determinant of our happiness and peace of mind. If we use our time judiciously and efficiently, we can become more successful. However, if we do not use our time appropriately, our productivity decreases. Inefficiency in managing our time may create problems. It leads to unfulfillment of our expectations and desired goals, which in turn can become a great source of stress. Therefore, managing time efficiently and effectively holds great significance.

Another important dimension with regard to utilizing our time is to have appropriate *balance* in our activities. We need to allocate adequate time for physical activities, mental enrichment, social interactions, and spiritual well being. All these dimensions are important spokes of a "holistic wheel" for harmony in life as shown in Figure 9.1.

One popular management principle, in the context of time management, is the **Pareto Principle**. According to this principle, most of the desired key results are obtained by only a few of our total activities. On the other hand, the majority of other activities generate only a few of the key results. Pareto estimated that this relationship was 20 to 80 percent in most situations; that is, 80 percent of the results would be derived from 20 percent of the objectives, whereas 80 percent of the objectives would yield only 20 percent of the results. Therefore, *priority*

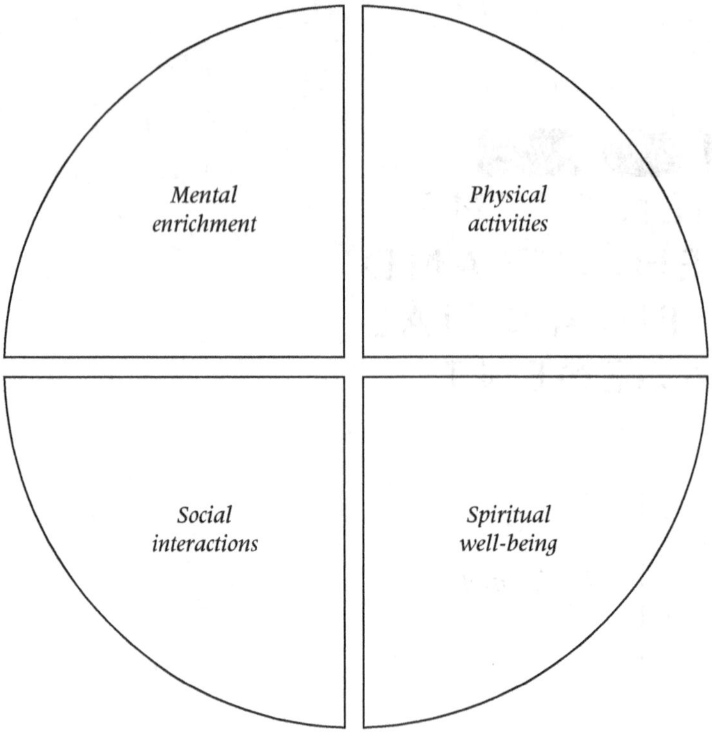
Mental enrichment
Physical activities
Social interactions
Spiritual well-being

Figure 9.1 "Holistic Wheel" of Harmony in Life

of effort may be given to those objectives identified as the *critical few* (Liebler, & McConnell, 2012). That means we should focus on urgent and important tasks. This approach of learning and practicing to prioritize our daily activities and tasks in order to optimize results will be the basis for our discussion on efficient time management.

manifestations of poor time management

Poor time management seems to be a universal problem. Studies on time management generally show that the majority of us, most of the time, admit to not managing our time very well and acknowledge that this failure creates stress in our lives. Some manifestations of poor time management are:

- Unfulfilled expectations
- Inability to be on time for appointments
- Hurrying to be on time
- Poor planning
- Inability to achieve desired objectives
- Tiredness and fatigue resulting from unplanned downtime
- Regret over missed deadlines
- Disappointments

- ○ Inadequate time for rest

- ○ Borrowing time from time slots for family, work, leisure, free time, or personal relationships

- ○ Constant feeling of being overwhelmed

- ○ Feeling of "too much going on"

- ○ Worrying about how to get things done

- ○ Inability to deliver goods on time

- ○ Insecure feelings about the future

- ○ Regrets about the past

Therefore, poor time management is an important source of stress and leads to negative harmful consequences. These undue negative consequences are self-inflicted and can be easily prevented if we understand, apply, and follow the basic principles of time management.

Self-understanding is a prerequisite to making any change, particularly in changing our behavior in relation to efficient time management (Januz & Jones, 1981). Therefore, before you proceed to learn about the basic principles of efficient time management, you need to gain an insight into your own behavior and find out whether managing time is a problem for you. This understanding will provide you with a benchmark as to where you can start your efforts at managing time efficiently and effectively. **Worksheet 9.1** (page 199) is designed to help you enhance this understanding. See also Box 9.1, Time Waster Personalities (page 192). Thoughts for Reflection 9.1, Barriers to Efficient Time Management (page 193), will help you to ponder some of the barriers that may be preventing you from managing your time efficiently.

approaches to time management

Time management has acquired greater significance in modern times. Never before in history has time management been given such importance. Present life has become much faster paced than in the past. Therefore, approaches for time management need to address current times. A plethora of ideas have been suggested for time management (Assagioli, 1973; Davis, Eshelman, & McKay, 2008; Eliot & Breo, 1989; Greenberg, 2010; Greenwald, 1973; Lakein, 1973; Levinson, 1990; Mackenzie, 1972; Smith, 1993; Swindoll, 1982). In essence, all these approaches to time management emphasize the need to *prioritize* our daily activities and implement a plan to achieve them. From a practical point of view, the basic technique consists of the following components:

- ○ Developing awareness about how one spends one's time

- ○ Setting long-term goals

- ○ Identifying short-term objectives to accomplish these goals

- ○ Establishing priorities

- ○ Concrete decision making about key priorities

- ○ Realistic scheduling and elimination of low priorities

BOX **9·1**

Time Waster Personalities

Brian Seaward (2012), in his book on managing stress, describes six personalities that can be classified as time wasters:

1. **Type A personality** characteristics are described in Chapter 1. On the surface, Type A personality people may appear to be organized and productive, but evidence points to the contrary. These people, in their pursuit for competition, tend to complete tasks in a hurry, spend time in hostility, and try to perform several tasks at one time, all of which amount to wasting time.

2. **Workaholics** tend to derive satisfaction from long work hours. In essence, these people tend to do trivial tasks in normal work hours and major projects after hours, do not use timesaving measures, and derive pleasure in working long hours, all of which amount to wasting time.

3. **Time jugglers** try to perform more than one thing at a time. Have you ever seen a person who is driving, using a cell phone, grabbing a sandwich, and soothing a child in the rear seat—all at the same time? These people tend to begin several tasks without reaching closure on any, miss out on important responsibilities, and spend more time than needed on tasks—thus making them time wasters.

4. **Procrastinators** apply diversion tactics and put off what needs to be done today. They tend to do *less difficult* tasks rather than *important* tasks, take a stab at the task but find an excuse to drift away from completing it, and knowingly do things other than the job at hand, all of which amount to wasting time.

5. **Perfectionists** are obsessed with carrying out every task to perfection. They get caught in detail, never see the big picture, are too hard on themselves and others, and perform the same task repeatedly, all of which add to wasting time.

6. **Lifestyle behavior trappers** have a hard time saying no. Since they have other people's agendas thrust upon them, they never make efforts at organizing their tasks. They look for gratification from others, and they end up wasting time.

○ Overcoming possible barriers

○ Implementing the plan of priorities to manage time efficiently

This basic technique of time management helps us in achieving our long-term goals as well as assists in accomplishing our daily activities. Developing a longer time horizon is important from a future perspective, while accomplishment of daily activities is important from a current perspective. Both these dimensions play an important role in preventing and reducing undue stress in our life. In this chapter, we focus on managing time with respect to accomplishing daily activities and tasks. The skills pertaining to setting goals and objectives are discussed in Chapter 10. One needs to remember that daily tasks and activities ought to be guided by establishing a vision, mission, and goals. Therefore, in this chapter we do not discuss what goals to set and how to define objectives in meeting those goals. We assume that goals have already been set, and from there we elaborate on a practical technique for managing time to accomplish daily activities and tasks. You may now complete **Worksheet 9.2** (page 202), which has been designed for this purpose. You also need to ponder Thoughts for Reflection 9.2, It Has Been Quite Some Time. . . (page 193), which will help you appreciate the

■ **Inability to Prioritize.** If we are not familiar with the basic principles of prioritization, do not have the necessary skills, or are not willing to prioritize, then any of these situations will act as a barrier to efficient time management. Prioritizing daily activities, short-term objectives, and long-term goals is central to efficient time management.

■ **Inability to Say No.** It is simply not possible to please everyone. Nor is it possible to please some people all the time. Therefore, the ability to say no to others if we want to say no, even if it may be somewhat displeasing, is a valuable practice in efficiently managing our time. This ability allows us to accomplish our goals and objectives and not become distracted.

■ **Imbalance in Life.** We may be neglecting or overindulging in some of our daily activities. We may be overactive physically while neglecting our mental enrichment. Or we may be socially active but have low levels of physical activity. Or we may be completely bankrupt spiritually. Or we

may be involved in too many mental activities, so we become isolated socially. We need balance in all areas of life.

■ **Too Many Improperly Planned Desires.** The mind is a very powerful source of generating desires. There is nothing wrong with having desires per se, but if we do not have a proper plan to accomplish these desires, then they do more harm than good. We need to select a few key desires, make a plan to achieve them, and work at the plan.

■ **Lack of Focus.** If we are not focused on our goals, we will most often spend our time on misdirected activities. We need to think and decide what we want to achieve and then make focused efforts in order to optimize the use of our time.

■ **Procrastination.** The habit of delaying accomplishment of any task to the very last minute is a serious barrier in efficient time management. Once we know what we need to do, we need to accomplish it as soon as possible.

It has been quite some time since I have noticed nature and its beauty around me. When was the last time I looked upon and pondered the blue, beautiful, magnanimous sky, the majestic snow-peaked mountains, the green thick forests, the bright shining sun, or other beauties of nature?

It has been even longer since I reflected on the daily intricate and seemingly small events around me. When was the last time I noticed a child's smile, a gesture of kindness by people around me, a token of appreciation, or other gifts of human love?

Rather, I have been too busy with daily hassles—meeting deadlines, fulfilling obligations, yielding to demands, and chasing desires. I have been either regretting

past events or worrying about future happenings.

■ Am I doing the right thing?

■ Am I using my time wisely?

■ Am I happy, content, and satisfied?

■ Do I have peace of mind?

Two issues seem apparent. First, I have not taken enough time for myself. Second, I have ignored the most important frontier, "the now!" I have not completely understood the true value of "today" and the importance of having time available for myself. I need to reflect and restore the inherent joy of having *time for myself now.*

- Set priorities.

- Adhere to established priorities.

- Avoid procrastination.

- Avoid gossip.

- Have a balance in types of activities.

- Avoid unnecessary socialization.

- Self-organize.

- Delegate tasks.

- Do not always seek perfection.

- Have faith in the ability of others.

- Overcome undue frustration.

- Simplify the tasks.

- Refuse when you would like to refuse.

- Have free time to reflect and plan.

- Think before doing.

- Do not overindulge in only pleasure-seeking activities.

- Make written lists of daily tasks to be done.

importance of having time for yourself and focusing on the present. Thoughts for Reflection 9.3 above provides some ideas on how you can save time.

sound financial management

Along with time management, another aspect of personal efficiency that requires attention is financial management. Just like time, money is a finite resource that needs to be wisely managed. Finances are a common source of stress, particularly for college students and especially from credit cards. According to a national survey, 83 percent of undergraduate students carry at least one credit card (Barrett, 2003). The survey further found that 21 percent of undergraduates who have credit cards have unpaid balances between $3,000 and $7,000. Most students usually incur these expenses during spring-break trips. If one takes a $1,000 trip and borrows money on a credit card with a 15.9 percent interest rate and makes only minimum payments, it will take 15 1/2 years to pay off the balance. The $1,000 trip turns into a $2,329 trip with the accumulated interest.

Credit cards are a very useful tool in our present-day world. One does not need to carry around large sums of money and can use credit cards for buying anything from groceries to appliances and other expensive items. If used judiciously, credit cards can be great assets. By "using judiciously," we mean paying off the credit card balance in full and on time every month and not carrying over any debt.

Oftentimes students are not able to manage their credit cards and run up enormous amounts of debt at an extremely high interest rate. High interest rates on credit cards result in spending large amounts of money just to pay the interest. Recent changes in legislation have made it difficult to easily get rid of credit card debt. Carrying such debt and the inability to pay off debt adversely affects one's credit rating and can cause financial stress. In addition to credit cards, there are other sources of financial stress for college students. Some of these include:

- Tuition costs

- Boarding and lodging expenses

- The cost of books

- Cell phone bills

- Travel costs, especially if away from home

- Study abroad, if interested

- Entertainment costs

- Emergency expenditures

Knowing about resources that can help pay for tuition and college costs is a step to improving financial management. Student grants, student loans, and personal resources are three options to explore.

Student grants are "free" money that is given to the student to cover college-related expenses. Grants can range from a few hundred dollars to thousands of dollars. A grant is not a loan and does not need to be paid back. Some grants are need-based and some are merit-based. There are four main sources of grants: (a) federal, (b) state, (c) college-specific, and (d) private. Examples of some current federal grants include Pell Grants, Federal Supplemental Opportunity Grants, Teacher Education Assistance for College and Higher Education (TEACH) Grants, Academic Competitiveness Grants (ACG), National Science and Mathematics Access to Retain Talent Grants (National SMART Grant), and Iraq and Afghanistan Service Grants. An online search for these grants can provide you with more details.

You must complete a Free Application for Federal Student Aid (FAFSA) application, available at http://fafsa.ed.gov to apply for federal grants. Likewise, several states provide grants to their residents and one can explore applying for those as well. Colleges typically provide several grants that can be tapped. Finally, there are private foundations that give grants, such as those offered by the Educational Employees Credit Union, GE Foundation, Baptist Memorial Health Care, Geological Society of America, and Harry S. Truman Scholarship Foundation. You can find out more about these grants from your financial aid administration office, from your friends, from college publications, and from Internet search.

Student loans are another way of funding college costs. There are two main types of student loans: (a) federal, and (b) private. Federal loans are distributed by the government and usually have lower rates while private loans are made by private entities such as banks. Federal loans typically need to start being repaid 6–9 months after graduation while private loans usually require repayment to begin right after graduation. If possible, you should try to satisfy your financial need with federal loans first before looking to private loans. Some loans are interest-free, some have low interest rates and others have high interest rates. Obviously, free or low interest rate lows are preferable to high interest rate ones, and you should try to satisfy financial need with those first before resorting to high interest rate loans.

If you have personal resources, then you can use those for college expenses as well. When using your own or your family's resources, it becomes even more important to plan the expenses and make a budget to utilize those resources.

Poor financial management can lead to financial stress. Financial stress often causes conditions like anxiety and depression. Financial stress can also adversely affect sleep, which in turn can affect cognitive abilities and one's ability to function effectively. Carrying debt also causes one to cut corners in spending for key areas such as health care or even basic necessities such as food and clothing. Thoughts for Reflection 9.4, Warning Signs of Too Much Debt on Credit Cards (page 196), provides a list of warning signs to identify when you have too much debt on credit cards.

WARNING SIGNS OF TOO MUCH DEBT ON CREDIT CARDS

If you have one or more of the following signs, you may be running too much debt on credit cards.

▪ You do not have any significant savings and use credit cards for purchases.

▪ You have not calculated the total amount of money you owe on credit cards.

▪ You make only the minimum monthly payment on credit cards.

▪ You are often late in paying your credit card bill.

▪ You are using several credit cards and one or more of those have reached the credit limit.

▪ You have been refused credit by a potential lender.

▪ You have a low credit score.

▪ You have started cutting corners on essentials.

▪ Despite the debt, you continue to use credit cards.

▪ You avoid talking about your financial situation.

We need to be cognizant of our spending habits and must aim at spending within our limits. We must create a monthly budget and adhere to it. Creating a budget is vital to keeping our "financial house" in order. In a budget, we show where the money is coming from and where the money is going so that we do not overspend and keep our debt to a minimum. **Worksheet 9.3** (page 207) helps enhance our awareness about our financial status and create a budget. Here are some reasons why we should create a financial inventory:

○ Tells us how much we are earning.

○ Tells us how much we are spending.

○ Shows us things on which we are spending money.

○ Identifies ways by which we can cut down costs and save money.

○ Helps us plan ahead of time how we are going to spend money.

○ Aligns our financial goals with our priorities and goals in life.

CHAPTER REVIEW

summary points

○ Time is a precious resource that needs to be managed efficiently and effectively.

○ We need to have appropriate balance in our physical activities, mental enrichment, social interactions, and spiritual well being.

○ According to Pareto's principle, most of our desired key results are obtained by only a few of our activities, while the majority of our activities generate only a few key results. Usually this ratio is 80:20.

○ Some manifestations of poor time management include unfulfilled expectations, inability to be on time for appointments, hurrying, disappointment, regrets, and so on.

○ Self-understanding is a prerequisite to efficient time management.

○ Barriers to efficient time management include the inability to prioritize, the inability to say no, imbalance in life, too many improperly planned desires, lack of focus, and procrastination.

○ Central to all approaches to time management is the understanding and practice of prioritization.

○ There are two important things for peace and happiness: having time for oneself and focusing on the present.

○ Just like time, money is also a finite resource that needs to be wisely managed.

○ Creating a budget is vital to keeping the financial house in order.

important terms defined

ABC list: A list that categorizes all tasks at any given time into high value (urgent and important), medium value (less urgent and less important), and low value (least urgent and least important).

budget: Monthly account of where the money is coming from and where the money is being spent.

Pareto Principle: A management principle that purports that 80 percent of the result is achieved by 20 percent of the objectives while 20 percent of the result is achieved by 80 percent of the objectives.

perfectionist: A person who is obsessed with carrying out any task in complete detail without any self-perceived errors.

procrastinator: A person who consciously, subconsciously, or unconsciously delays completion of any given task at hand.

time juggler: A person who tries to perform more than one task at a time.

Type A personality: A person who is characterized by a hurrying nature, competitive zeal, dominating nature, and fast pace of life.

workaholic: A person who derives satisfaction from working long hours and is habituated or addicted to this way of life to a point that it starts affecting his or her personal life.

websites to explore

PERSONAL TIME MANAGEMENT FOR BUSY MANAGERS

www.ee.ed.ac.uk/~gerard/Management/

This website hosts an article by British author Gerard Blair in which he introduces several tips for effective time management for busy managers.

■ Visit the website, read the article, reflect, and write about any one tip that is useful in your personal life.

RANDY PAUSCH'S TIPS FOR TIME MANAGEMENT

www.alice.org/Randy/timetalk.htm

This website provides the "time talk" by Randy Pausch, given at Carnegie Mellon University.

- Closely examine the photographs on the website. What is one thing you learned, and how will you apply that on your study table?

TIME MANAGEMENT

www.mindtools.com/pages/main/newMN_HTE.htm

This website provides tips for time management.

- Visit the website, read the information, reflect, and write about any one tip that is useful in your personal life.

VIRTUAL PAMPHLET COLLECTION—TIME MANAGEMENT

http://counseling.uchicago.edu/page/virtual-pamphlet-collection-time-management

This website of the University of Chicago Student Counseling and Resource Service has a compilation of various virtual pamphlets from different universities on time management.

- Review this website and navigate the links. Which pamphlet did you like most and why?

Enhancing Awareness of How You Spend Your Time

Sit down, relax, and respond to the following questions, recalling the past week as best you can. There are no correct or incorrect answers. These questions are based on your recollection, and the more accurately you can recall events, the better your assessment will be. This worksheet will enhance your awareness about how you are using your time.

1. In the past week, were you late for any appointment(s)?

   _____ Yes _____ No _____ Not sure

   If yes, how many times? _____ out of _____ times.

   What percentage is this? _____

2. In the past week, did you miss breakfast, lunch, or supper in order to be on time for some task?

   _____ Yes _____ No _____ Not sure

   If yes, how many times? _____ out of 21 times.

   What percentage is this? _____

3. In the past week, did you do something that would be considered a waste of time? Think about each day during the past week, and count the number of hours per day that you wasted.

   _____ Less than 2 hours _____ 2 to 4 hours _____ More than 4 hours

4. In the past week, did you miss any deadlines at work or any other personal obligations? How many deadlines or obligations did you miss?

   _____ None _____ 1 _____ 2 or more

5. For the past week, total the number of hours you slept each day. Divide the total by seven to come up with a daily average for the week.

   _____ Less than 8 hours _____ 8–10 hours _____ More than 10 hours

6. For the past week, total the number of hours you spent each day on work (be sure to count hours spent at school as work). Divide the total by seven to come up with a daily average for the week.

   _____ Less than 8 hours _____ 8–10 hours _____ More than 10 hours

7. For the past week, total the number of hours you spent each day on personal hygiene. Divide the total by seven to come up with a daily average for the week.

   _____ Less than 60 minutes _____ 60–90 minutes _____ More than 90 minutes

(continued)

Enhancing Awareness of How You Spend Your Time *(cont'd)*

8. For the past week, total the number of hours you spent each day on preparing and eating meals. Divide the total by seven to come up with a daily average for the week.

   _____ Less than 3 hours _____ 3–4 hours _____ More than 4 hours

9. For the past week, total the number of hours each day that you consider free time. Divide the total by seven to come up with a daily average for the week.

   _____ Less than 2 hours _____ 2–3 hours _____ More than 3 hours

10. In the past week, how many times did you procrastinate for a task that you were doing?

   _____ None _____ 1 _____ 2 or more

FEEDBACK ON WORKSHEET 9.1

1. During the past week if you were on time for 80 percent or more of your appointments, you are doing an excellent job with time management (give yourself 2 points); 60–80 percent means there is room for improvement (give yourself 1 point); and if you were late for more than 40 percent of the time, then you need to diligently apply the skills described in this chapter (give yourself no points).

2. If you missed no meals, then you are doing an excellent job with time management (give yourself 2 points). If you missed up to 3 meals, then there is room for improvement (give yourself 1 point). If you missed more than 3 meals, you need to diligently apply the time management skills described in this chapter (give yourself no points).

3. In the past week, if you wasted less than 2 hours, then you are doing an excellent job with time management (give yourself 2 points). However, if you wasted 2–4 hours, then there is room for improvement (give yourself 1 point). If you wasted more than 4 hours, then you need to diligently apply the time management skills described in this chapter (give yourself no points).

4. If you did not miss any deadlines at work or any other personal obligations, then you are doing an excellent job with time management (give yourself 2 points). However, if you missed one deadline, there is room for improvement (give yourself 1 point); and if you missed two or more deadlines, you need to diligently apply the time management skills described in this chapter (give yourself no points).

5. If you marked less than 8 hours or more than 10 hours of sleep per day, give yourself no points. You need to diligently apply the time management skills described in this chapter. If you marked 8 to 10 hours, you are on the right track and you can give yourself 2 points.

6. If you marked less than 8 hours or more than 10 hours of work per day, give yourself no points. You need to diligently apply the time management skills described in this chapter. If you marked 8 to 10 hours, you are on the right track and you can give yourself 2 points. In the United States, it is customary to consider 40 hours per week full-time employment, and it is the standard duration for work time per week for most healthy people. Most people spend additional time preparing for these work hours—sometimes on weekends—so the range of 40 to 50 hours per week is considered an ideal amount of time spent on work. Too little work yields too much free time and potential for stress. Too much time spent on work reduces free time, thus adding to stress.

7. If you marked less than 60 minutes or more than 90 minutes of personal hygiene per day, give yourself no points. You need to diligently apply the skills described in this chapter. If you marked 60 to 90 minutes, you are on the right track and you can give yourself 2 points. Personal hygiene includes several different activities, such as brushing teeth, using the restroom, washing hands, taking showers, applying makeup, dressing, and so on. Most people spend 60 to 90 minutes on these activities. If you are spending less time on hygiene, then you are compromising on some important activities, which can add stress to your life. If you are overindulging in these activities, then you will have less time for other activities in your life, which will prevent balance and cause stress.

8. If you marked less than 3 hours or more than 4 hours for meals per day, give yourself no points. You need to become proficient in this aspect of time management. If you marked 3 to 4 hours, you are on the right track and you can give yourself 2 points.

9. If you marked less than 2 hours or more than 3 hours of free time per day, give yourself no points. You need to become more proficient in applying the skills described in this chapter. If you marked 2 to 3 hours, you are on the right track and you can give yourself 2 points.

10. In the past week if you did not procrastinate at all, then you are doing an excellent job with time management (give yourself 2 points). However, if you procrastinated once, there is room for improvement (give yourself 1 point); and if you procrastinated two or more times, you need to diligently apply the time management skills described in this chapter (give yourself no points).

If your overall score is a perfect 20, then continue doing what you are already doing with regard to time management. Congratulations on a perfect score! If your score is between 15 and 19, you likely need to improve in one or more areas of time management. If your score is less than 14, you will need to diligently apply the skills discussed in this chapter, as time management is certainly an area needed for your growth.

Practical Steps to Time Management

Complete the following worksheet to set priorities for your daily and long-term activities.

STEP 1. DEVELOPING AWARENESS ABOUT HOW YOU ARE CURRENTLY SPENDING YOUR TIME

Worksheet 9.1 (page 199) has already provided you with some insights. Now you can summarize those findings in a chronological and meaningful sequence in the space provided:

PAST 1 WEEK:

Activities desired	Activities performed

PAST 1 MONTH:

Activities desired	Activities performed

Practical Steps to Time Management *(cont'd)*

PAST 1 YEAR:

Activities desired	Activities performed

A comparison between the activities desired and performed will provide you with an understanding of the gap that exists and needs to be filled.

STEP 2. LIST OF DESIRED ACTIVITIES

Now, make a comprehensive, chronological list of the activities that you want to accomplish.

TODAY:

_____

_____

_____

_____

_____

_____

_____

_____

_____

_____

(continued)

Practical Steps to Time Management *(cont'd)*

WITHIN THE NEXT WEEK:

_____

_____

_____

_____

_____

_____

_____

WITHIN THE NEXT MONTH:

_____

_____

_____

_____

_____

_____

_____

_____

WITHIN THE NEXT YEAR:

_____

_____

_____

_____

_____

_____

_____

Practical Steps to Time Management *(cont'd)*

STEP 3. ESTABLISHING PRIORITIES

Ask yourself, "What is the best use of my time right now?" Having reflected upon this question, you need to classify all desired activities into an **ABC list:** A—high value (activities that need to be done absolutely and immediately), B—medium value (activities that need to be accomplished as soon as possible), and C—low value (activities that need to be done at some time or may even be ignored).

	Category A	Category B	Category C
TODAY:			
WITHIN THE NEXT WEEK:			
WITHIN THE NEXT MONTH:			
WITHIN THE NEXT YEAR:			

(continued)

Practical Steps to Time Management *(cont'd)*

STEP 4. REASSESSING PRIORITIES

Every day, before going to bed, you need to reassess the priorities set in Step 3 and see which ones remain unfulfilled. You should identify any obstacles or barriers that may have been responsible. Then you need to make necessary changes. You can record your observations in the space provided:

_____

_____

_____

_____

_____

_____

_____

FEEDBACK ON WORKSHEET 9.2

This worksheet should have helped you prioritize your daily activities as well as possible activities in the near future. You need to make focused efforts at achieving activities listed in category A. After having accomplished the activities in category A, you need to proceed to complete the activities listed in category B. Only after accomplishing tasks in categories A and B should you look at tasks in category C—even though they may appear to be simple and easy. You should not be lured by this simplicity, and you should focus only on the importance of the activities.

WORKSHEET 9.3

This worksheet is available online at www.pearsonhighered.com/romas.

Enhancing Awareness About
Financial Status and Creating a Budget

Seek out a quiet place and complete the following worksheet. In order to complete this worksheet, you will need your bank statements, monthly pay stubs from all employers, details of investment accounts, details of retirement accounts, recent utility bills, rent or mortgage payment records, credit card bills, and a calculator.

Date: _____

A. SOURCES OF INCOME (MONTHLY):

1. Employer #1 (net monthly income after taxes and other deductions):

   $_____

2. Employer #2 (net monthly income after taxes and other deductions):

   $_____

3. Employer #3 (net monthly income after taxes and other deductions):

   $_____

4. All other employers (net monthly income): $_____

5. Other sources of monthly income (such as interest income, money from parents, etc.):

   $_____

6. Total monthly income (1 + 2 + 3 + 4 + 5): $_____

B. SAVINGS BALANCES:

7. Savings account(s): $_____

8. Investment accounts: $_____

9. Retirement accounts: $_____

10. Total savings (7 + 8 + 9): $_____

11. Goal for monthly savings:

    a Savings account(s): $_____

    b Investment account(s): $_____

    c Retirement account(s): $_____

    d Total (a + b + c): $_____

C. FIXED EXPENSES (MONTHLY):

12. Mortgage/Rent: $_____

13. Car payment: $_____

14. Auto insurance: $_____

(continued)

Enhancing Awareness About
Financial Status and Creating a Budget *(cont'd)*

15. Cable service: $_____

16. Internet service: $_____

17. Trash pickup: $_____

18. Other: $_____

19. Total fixed expenses (12 + 13 + 14 + 15 + 16 + 17 + 18): $_____

D. VARIABLE EXPENSES (MONTHLY):

Average the last 3 months or last 12 months, if data is available; otherwise make the best possible guess:

20. Groceries: $_____

21. Electric: $_____

22. Gas: $_____

23. Water: $_____

24. Sewage: $_____

25. Gasoline: $_____

26. Telephone: $_____

27. Eating out: $_____

28. Entertainment: $_____

29. Clothes: $_____

30. Gifts: $_____

31. Health care: $_____

32. School expenses (tuition, books, etc.): $_____

33. Credit cards: $_____

34. Other: $_____

35. Total variable expenses (20 + 21 + 22 + 23 + 24 + 25 + 26 + 27 + 28 + 29 + 30 + 31 + 32 + 33 + 34):

$_____

E. TOTAL EXPENSES (MONTHLY):

36. Sum up 19 + 35: $_____

Enhancing Awareness About
Financial Status and Creating a Budget *(cont'd)*

F. INCOME — EXPENSES:

37. Subtract 36 from 6: $_____

G. DEBTS:

38. Mortgage (amount remaining): $_____

39. Credit card #1 _____ : $_____

40. Credit card #2 _____ : $_____

41. Credit card #3 _____ : $_____

42. Credit card #4 _____ : $_____

43. Credit card #5 _____ : $_____

44. Other credit cards _____ : $_____

45. Student loans: $_____

46. Other debt: $_____

47. Credit card debt (39 + 40 + 41 + 42 + 43 + 44): $_____

48. Other debt (38 + 45 + 46): $_____

FEEDBACK ON WORKSHEET 9.3

If you have a positive number in item 37, you are doing a good job managing your monthly expenditures. You can also start saving more money and increase your goals in item 11. It is never too early to start saving for retirement. If the number in item 37 is a negative number, then you are in financial trouble. You must look at cutting your expenses and increasing your income. Go over the list of expenses and see which items you can reduce or totally eliminate without compromising the basic necessities. Also look carefully for ways to improve your income.

Now look at item 47. If this is a positive number, then you are likely paying a very high interest rate on this sum of money. This debt should be paid off as soon as possible. Make a definitive plan to pay this debt as soon as feasible and do not incur any more expenses on your credit cards. If you have savings, you may want to use some of that money to pay down this high interest debt. You may also consider taking another job to pay off this debt as soon as possible. Your goal for item 47 must be a zero that means you are paying off your credit card balance every month.

Review this worksheet on a monthly basis. After the first month take a moment to compare your actual expenses versus what you had estimated for the budget. This comparison will show you how accurate you were and where you may need to make modifications.

references and further readings

Assagioli, R. (1973). *The act of will*. New York: Viking Press.

Barrett, J. (2003). Excessive credit card use causes student debt woes. *Young Money*. Retrieved from http://www.youngmoney.com/credit_debt/get_out_of_debt/021007_03.

Burke, C. R., Hall, D. R., & Hawley, D. (1986). *Living with stress*. Clackamas, OR: Wellsource.

Davis, M., Eshelman, E. R., & McKay, M. (2008). *The relaxation and stress reduction workbook* (6th ed.). Oakland, CA: New Harbinger.

Eliot, R. S., & Breo, D. L. (1989). *Is it worth dying for? How to make stress work for you—not against you* (rev. ed.) (p. 216). New York: Bantam.

Greenberg, J. S. (2010). *Comprehensive stress management* (12th ed.). Boston: McGraw-Hill.

Greenwald, H. (1973). *Direct decision therapy*. San Diego: EDITS.

Hanson, P. G. (1986). *The joy of stress*. New York: Andrews and McNeal.

Januz, L. R., & Jones, S. K. (1981). *Time management for executives*. New York: Scribner.

Lakein, A. (1973). *How to get control of your time and your life*. New York: Signet.

Levinson, J. C. (1990). *The ninety-minute hour*. New York: Dutton.

Liebler,, J. G.., & McConnell, C. R. (2012). *Management principles for health professionals* (6th ed.). Sudbury, MA: Jones & Bartlett.

Mackenzie, A. (1972). *The time trap*. New York: AMACOM.

Rice, P. L. (1999). *Stress and health* (3rd ed.). Belmont, CA: Wadsworth.

Seaward, B. L. (2012). *Managing stress: Principles and strategies for health and well being* (7th ed.). Boston: Jones and Bartlett.

Smith, J. C. (1993). *Creative stress management: The 1–2–3 cope system*. Englewood Cliffs, NJ: Prentice Hall.

Swindoll, C. R. (1982). *Strengthening your grip: How to live confidently in an aimless world*. Dallas: Word.

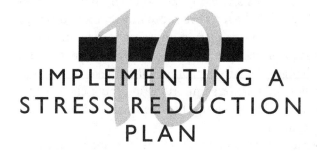

IMPLEMENTING A STRESS REDUCTION PLAN

"Work on a plan; then the plan will work on you."

importance of implementing a plan

Any intention—however noble it may be, any plan—however well conceived it may be, any desire—however chaste it may be, unless implemented cannot produce the necessary results. We need to implement our intentions, plans, and desires in order to obtain the necessary results. The purpose of this workbook is to provide practical suggestions toward preventing, reducing, and managing the harmful and negative consequences of stress in our daily lives, thus enabling us to effectively manage changes that are an inevitable part of life. These practical suggestions, if not implemented in our lives, are meaningless. We need to make conscious efforts at integrating these suggestions into our daily activities. These efforts will foster positive health and promote our well being.

The starting point in the process of implementation is to take stock of the resources that are available to us. In implementing a stress reduction plan, a prerequisite is to have self-motivation. Unless and until we are motivated to bring about change in our lives, nobody can force us to make that change. We need to be committed. We need to have faith in ourselves and the techniques that we are going to implement. We also need to be aware of what needs to be changed (Romas & Zenga, 2001).

Another prerequisite for success is the degree of changeability in what we intend to change in our behavior. This changeability varies from individual to individual and is person-specific. For example, applying relaxation techniques may be more changeable for some of us but difficult for others who have a more rigid lifestyle, or applying anxiety-coping techniques may be more changeable for some of us while others may find it more difficult, and so on. From a practical point of view, we need to prioritize and put our efforts into those behavior patterns that are changeable and important (Green & Kreuter, 2005). We need to identify for ourselves, on our own, which behaviors are less changeable and which behaviors are more changeable, and which behaviors are more important and which behaviors are less important. The behaviors that are more important and more changeable need to be our first priority. Then, we need to alter behaviors that are more important but less changeable. After accomplishing these two sets of behaviors, we can tackle behaviors that are less important and more changeable. Behaviors that are less important and less changeable need to be ignored. This aspect is presented later in the chapter.

After having this requisite motivation and conditioning, we need to identify friends, co-workers, family members, associates, and others who can help us in our efforts to implement our stress reduction plan. We need to take them into confidence and share our plan. We need to solicit their support in helping us adhere to the plan. They will provide us with the necessary mental, emotional, and social support that will help keep us from deviating from our decisions. We also need to procure any special accessories or equipment required for implementing the desired set of behaviors. For example, for a cross-country skiing program, we need to have ski gear, appropriate clothing, conditioning, and a location.

We also need to make definitive time allocations for implementing our plan. This requirement will entail scheduling the activities for desired behaviors (as suggested in several worksheets throughout this workbook) into our daily plan, however busy we may be. We need to allocate regular blocks of time for implementing techniques for prevention, reduction, and management of stress.

Finally, we need to make this stress reduction plan fit into our overall scheme of life. To do so, we need to have clarity about where we want to be, or in other words—what our goal is. We also need to clearly know how we will achieve this goal, that is, which objectives will lead us to that goal.

Such planning has been shown to improve our coping skills with everyday stressors as well as chronic stressors. Chris Kleinke (2002) uses the basic framework of goal setting for coping with a myriad of situations such as failure, loneliness, loss, aging, pain, illness, and injury. Hopefully, you will find these planning techniques very helpful.

stages of change

In making a plan for changing stress-related behaviors, we need to understand that, when making this change, we progress through several stages. Since the 1980s, James Prochaska and his colleagues have developed a model popularly known as the "transtheoretical model" or the "stages of change model" to explain these stages systematically (2008). See Figure 10.1. According to this model, with regard to any behavior, a person begins in precontemplation, or is not aware that he or she needs to make the change and has no intention to change over the next 6 months. The second stage is contemplation, in which the person starts thinking about making a change regarding the behavior and wants to make the change within the next 6 months. The third stage is preparation, in which the person intends to take action within the next 30 days and has begun taking some behavioral steps in that direction. The fourth step is action, in which the person has initiated the changed behavior but has not done so continuously for 6 months. The final stage is maintenance, in which the person has been performing the desired behavior for more than 6 months continuously. After you have read this workbook, we are sure that

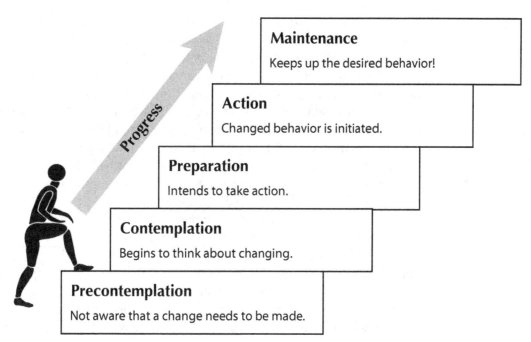

Figure 10.1 James Prochaska's Stages of Change Model

you would have progressed to at least the contemplation or preparation stages and would be ready to enter into the action and maintenance stages concerning one or more specific areas of stress management.

The stages of change model has been applied to a variety of health behaviors in a number of settings (Sharma & Romas, 2012). This model has been useful in helping people change behaviors. The model also elaborates on the role of self-efficacy and decisional balance in initiation of behavior change. Self-efficacy is the behavior-specific confidence that a person has in his or her abilities to perform a given behavior at any moment. It can be built by performing the behavior in small steps. In this workbook, you have learned the small steps for stress management-related behaviors. You must apply these steps to gain mastery of the behavior slowly over time. In developing self-efficacy, it is also essential to overcome temptations or urges to engage in a specific habit under difficult situations. Reducing stress, controlling cravings, and having positive social situations can achieve self-efficacy. The decisional balance is about having an understanding that the pros, or benefits, of changing outweigh the cons, or costs, of changing. Only when we are convinced that the pros of behavior change are more worthwhile than the cons will we initiate the behavior change. We should try to make a list of all the benefits of the change that we propose to make. With this understanding we are ready to develop our specific goals and objectives.

determining goals, objectives, and targets

GOAL SETTING

Goals are the total of projections of our long-term plans. Goals are an indication of what we want to accomplish in our lives. Goals signify a mission, an ambition, a purpose, and overall aim in life. These goals are oftentimes broad in nature. We need to identify goals for ourselves in different spheres of life, namely *personal, professional, social, financial,* and *spiritual.* An example of a personal goal could be achieving personal happiness and peace of mind; an example of a professional goal could be achieving a certain position within an organization; an example of a social goal could be marital contentment; an example of a financial goal could be establishing a solid savings plan; and an example of a spiritual goal could be achieving world peace. Attaining goals within these spheres is important from the perspective of deriving balance, harmony, and satisfaction in life. If any of these components are missing, then life will not be holistic, and thus, complete happiness will elude us. A person without goals is also likely to have greater stress in life because of undirected, aimless efforts.

Goal analysis or *goal setting* is a procedure useful in helping us describe the meaning of what we want to achieve in terms of attitude and understanding (Mager, 1972). The concept of setting goals implies that it is not necessarily important to achieve things in the "right way" but to do the "right things." An understanding of what these "right things" are for us is central to goal setting. The sense of direction in our activities is essentially an internally driven behavior. A number of theories have been presented to explain this behavior. One of the most popular theories in psychology, Maslow's *hierarchy of needs theory* on motivation (Maslow, 1954, 1962), identifies the following five levels of needs:

1. Physiological (food, clothing, shelter, sex, and so on)

2. Security and safety (protection from physical and emotional harm)

3. Love, affection, belonging, and social acceptance

4. Self-esteem (internal factors such as self-respect, autonomy, and achievement; and external factors such as status, recognition, attention, and so on)

5. Self-actualization (to achieve one's maximum potential)

According to Maslow, a person progresses from lower-level needs, such as physiological and security and safety, to higher-level needs, such as self-esteem and self-actualization, during the course of one's lifetime. Maslow hypothesized that the ultimate goal in life for all human beings was to reach self-actualization. According to this theory, it is important to accomplish a lower level of need before proceeding to the next level.

However, later research led to a modification of this theory. Clayton Alderfer (1969) revised this concept and presented an *ERG theory.* ERG is an acronym of the words *existence, relatedness,* and *growth.* These are the three groups of core needs. *Existence* is concerned with basic material requirements (same as Maslow's physiological and safety needs); *relatedness* is similar to Maslow's love need and the external component of Maslow's self-esteem classification; and *growth* is similar to the internal self-esteem component and self-actualization of Maslow's theory. However, the key features that differentiate this ERG theory from Maslow's theory are: (1) More than one level of need may be operative at the same time, and (2) if gratification of a higher-level need is blocked, then the desire to satisfy a lower-level need is increased. The ERG theory has greater scientific validation (Robbins & Judge, 2008).

This basic understanding of motivation is important in enabling us to set our goals. We need to be conscious about the "level of need" operating within our mind at any time. We also need to understand that the ultimate goal in life is to achieve our maximum potential or self-actualization.

ESTABLISHING OBJECTIVES

Objectives can be defined as concerted, directed, and focused step-by-step efforts to achieve goals. Objectives are more precise than goals and represent smaller steps. Some of the attributes in establishing objectives are as follows:

○ Precise (clear and not vague statements directed toward goal accomplishment)

○ Made to include a determined time frame (for example: one month, one year)

○ Realistic (accomplishable within available time frame and resources)

○ Sequenced (logical flow of steps leading to reaching the goal)

○ Written (to enhance clarity and provide a documented record for future reference)

○ Proactive (described by action verbs and self-driven)

○ Measurable (changes can be monitored in concrete terms)

○ Behaviorally oriented (imply specific behavior changes that need to be accomplished)

EXAMPLE OF AN OBJECTIVE

I will be able to identify one irrational belief responsible for causing my work-related anxiety, within the next week, *and achieve proficiency in practicing* progressive muscle relaxation *(PMR), as evinced by a feeling of relaxation by my body, after 10 minutes of daily practice, performed after coming home from work.*

This objective may appear to be slightly verbose, but we have attempted to explain most of the attributes within this example. While formulating objectives for ourselves, only we can be the best judge of the criteria that need inclusion and the criteria that can be excluded.

DECIDING TARGETS

To achieve practical accomplishment of goals and objectives, we need to perform a number of day-to-day activities. Identifying these daily activities in advance is important in planning. This process is known as deciding targets. **Targets** are things you do every day to advance you toward your goal. An example of a target would be *"I will, at 6:00 p.m., after returning from work, perform progressive muscle relaxation."*

Now, with the help of **Worksheet 10.1** (page 220), you can set goals and establish objectives. **Worksheet 10.2** (page 223) has been designed to prioritize your objectives. **Worksheet 10.3** (page 224) will help you decide upon daily targets in order to prioritize objectives. Record your daily targets for different objectives either on photocopies of Worksheet 10.3 or a separate blank sheet of paper.

Thoughts for Reflection 10.1, Points to Ponder (page 216), will help you ponder some ideas to keep in mind before setting goals and establishing objectives. Box 10.1, Eastern Views on Obtaining Results (page 216), presents some Eastern thoughts on obtaining results.

social support

Each of us has a set of social relationships. Some of these social relationships are merely people who we know casually. These relationships are called *social networks* (Heaney & Israel, 2002). All members of the social network may or may not be

BOX 10·1

Eastern Views on Obtaining Results

Most of our stress is due to expecting specific results from our actions. We are not sure what results we will get, and this uncertainty is often a source of fear, anxiety, and other forms of stress. According to Eastern philosophy, results are bound to follow any action. This is the basic law of nature: the law of cause and effect. The uncertain nature of results is also mandatory. According to this theory, results depend on the following three aspects:

- *Effort.* No result can occur without an *effort* on our part. *Effort* is the first and foremost step toward obtaining results.

- *Direction.* If our *effort* lacks an appropriate *direction*, then we will not be able to obtain the necessary results. Therefore, having a *direction*, or focus, is important to achieving success in our *effort*.

- *Unknown factor.* Even after applying an *effort* in an appropriate *direction*, success sometimes does not come. Such failures are due to the unknown factor

that is operating in the universal system of law. Religious-minded people refer to this as God; scientists attribute it to probability and chance. Without being unduly concerned about the semantics, the basic fact remains that we need to acknowledge and accept this inherent phenomenon. We then need to strengthen our mind and not be upset if the results do not go our way.

The only aspects over which we have control are *effort* and *direction.* Having applied our *effort* and having done so in the right *direction*, we need to think no further. We need to develop an attitude of bearing whatever the results may be. If they are good, we need to be thankful to the unknown; if they are not to our expectation, we need to think about what went wrong, how we can rectify anything, if at all, and accept the result with fortitude and grace. If the result has been negative, we also need to think about changing our *effort* and *direction*—that is, the behavior—if it is faulty.

**POINTS TO
PONDER**

Goal setting and establishing objectives …

… are not wishful thinking or daydreaming.

… are positive and proactive.

… are an individual activity that no one else can do for us.

… are not something to make us regret the past or worry about for the future.

… are a powerful tool for success in life.

… are an act of discipline.

… are effective for reducing stress, managing change, and promoting health.

---

helpful to us. However, some members are helpful to us and provide positive aid or assistance, especially during moments of crises. These members are known as **social support** (Heaney & Israel, 2008). Social support is a key factor that protects the individual from negative consequences of stress (Cassel, 1976; Heaney & Israel, 2008). Social support is always perceived by the sender to be positive and is intended to help in modifying the thoughts and actions of the receiver. House (1981) has identified four kinds of social support: (1) *emotional*, which includes expressions of love, empathy, caring, and trust; (2) *instrumental*, which includes tangible aid or

Let me make a promise to myself, for my own good, that …

… I will make an effort to practice what I have learned.

… I will be disciplined and proactive in my approach.

… I will remain optimistic and positive about life.

… I will have faith in myself, my goals, and the techniques I have learned.

… I will be enthusiastic and implement my plans with zeal.

… I will wear a cheerful countenance at all times and greet everyone around me with a smile.

… I will bless everyone around me, even if they may appear to be my enemies.

… I will devote my time to self-improvement—so much so that I will have no time to find mistakes in others.

… I will have no unrealistic expectation from people and situations around me.

… I will try to understand more often than I try to be understood.

… I will not allow worry over the future to overpower me and past events disturb my peace.

… I will be relaxed, happy, and content in my disposition with the present.

service; (3) *informational*, which includes advice, suggestions, and information; and (4) *appraisal*, which includes feedback for self-evaluation. These days a lot of college students and others are finding social support through interaction on social networking sites such as Facebook. In later years of college life, Facebook is particularly important in providing social support and well being to students (Kalpidou, Costin, & Morris, 2011). **Worksheet 10.4** (page 225) is designed for you to reflect on your sources of social support, and **Worksheet 10.5** (page 227) is about how to enhance the effectiveness of your social support. Take some time to reflect and complete these two worksheets before proceeding further.

finding the best techniques that suit your goals

All of us are different entities in ourselves. Our personalities, biological constitution, behaviors, values, attitudes, and beliefs are unique. Likewise, our goals are also bound to be unique and personal. There may be a similarity of pattern in our attributes and goals with other individuals, but ultimately this set of attributes that each of us has is unique and specific in itself. Therefore, as we have seen, it is important to identify stress management and reduction techniques that suit this uniqueness in our individuality and goals.

Worksheet 10.6 (page 228) is designed to provide you with an opportunity to identify and practice stress management and reduction techniques that suit your goals and "fit" your own unique individuality. These techniques, if practiced with *regularity* and *commitment*, are bound to produce beneficial results in achieving your goals.

Thoughts for Reflection 10.2, Promise to Myself, above, will help you reinforce a sense of commitment in order to keep up with the plan you decide upon.

toward a stress-free life

This workbook has provided you with techniques for preventing, reducing, and managing stress in your life. It is never too late to implement and practice these techniques regularly to obtain beneficial results. These results can be maximized if you incorporate these techniques within your daily life at a young age. Therefore, you should enter into an *agreement* with yourself to attain regularity by implementing the stress reduction plan in your life. If you attain this regularity for a continuous period of at least one year, it will become fully etched within your lifestyle. To achieve this continuity, you may reward yourself periodically with some tangible, self-decided rewards or incentives. **Worksheet 10.7** (page 231) is designed to help you with this objective.

Another helpful way to ensure this regularity is through social networking or building social support. Social networking also contributes to managing your stress directly. You need to identify a close group of people who are available for listening empathically to your views and concerns, who can help clarify questions, and who are willing to challenge you to grow if and when needed. Associating with such people helps prevent, reduce, and manage stress in your life. Finally, we emphasize that by regularly practicing selected techniques identified through this workbook you can effectively manage your stress.

CHAPTER REVIEW

summary points

- ○ Implementation of a plan is central for success.

- ○ Self-motivation and degree of changeability are prerequisites for implementing a plan.

- ○ The behaviors that are more important and more changeable deserve your first priority in implementation.

- ○ You need to take stock of all your resources before you implement a plan. This process includes soliciting help from people close to you and obtaining necessary material resources.

- ○ Goals are an indication of what you want to accomplish. They cover five different spheres of life: personal, professional, social, financial and spiritual.

- ○ Goal analysis or goal setting helps you describe the meaning of what you want to achieve in terms of attitude and understanding.

- ○ Maslow's hierarchy of needs theory for motivation identifies five levels of needs: physiological, security, love, self-esteem, and self-actualization.

- ○ Alderfer's ERG theory describes the core needs as existence, relatedness, and growth.

- ○ Objectives can be defined as concerted, directed, and focused step-by-step efforts for achieving goals.

- Some attributes in establishing objectives include precision, a determined time frame, and being realistic, sequenced, proactive, measurable, and behaviorally oriented.

- Deciding targets includes planning for the various day-to-day activities required in accomplishing goals and objectives.

- According to Eastern philosophy, success in any enterprise depends upon effort, direction, and an unknown factor.

- Regular practice of techniques described in this workbook will help you prevent, reduce, and manage your stress.

important terms defined

goal: A total of all projections or long-term plans. Goals signify an overall aim in life.

objectives: A concerted, directed, and focused step-by-step effort to achieve a goal. Objectives are precise, include a time frame, are realistic, are sequenced, use action verbs, and are measurable.

social support: The positive aid, either tangible or intangible, that is exchanged through social relationships and interpersonal transactions.

targets: Anything that a person does in everyday life to advance toward his or her goals.

websites to explore

GOAL SETTING

www.about-goal-setting.com/

This website, from a private organization, is about goal setting.

- Visit this website and complete a 20-minute tutorial.

SOCIAL ANXIETY SUPPORT GROUP

www.socialanxietysupport.com/

This website provides structured interactive forums and special programs to help those who suffer from social anxiety disorder (social phobia).

- Visit this website and peruse the cartoons or chat in one of the forums. Summarize your reactions.

TEN STEPS TO GETTING WHAT YOU WANT IN LIFE

www.gems4friends.com/goals/

This is the website of a private organization.

- Go through the ten steps. Did this reflection make sense in your life?

Determining Goals and Objectives

Seek out a quiet place to complete this worksheet. Write out an optimum number of goals and objectives—that is, not have too few or too many of each. It is also important to write these out. You need to periodically reexamine, reassess, and redefine your goals and objectives.

DATE: _____

A. SETTING GOALS

Personal goal:

_____

_____

_____

Professional goal:

_____

_____

_____

Social goal:

_____

_____

_____

Financial goal:

_____

_____

_____

Spiritual goal:

_____

_____

_____

Determining Goals and Objectives *(cont'd)*

B. ESTABLISHING OBJECTIVES

Objectives for personal goals:

_____

_____

_____

_____

_____

_____

_____

Objectives for professional goals:

_____

_____

_____

_____

_____

_____

_____

_____

Objectives for social goals:

_____

_____

_____

_____

_____

_____

_____

(continued)

Determining Goals and Objectives *(cont'd)*

Objectives for financial goals:

_____

_____

_____

_____

_____

_____

_____

Objectives for spiritual goals:

_____

_____

_____

_____

_____

_____

_____

WORKSHEET 10.2

This worksheet is available online at www.pearsonhighered.com/romas.

Prioritizing Your Objectives

Now prioritize your objectives from all five-goal categories:

	More Important	Less Important
More Changeable		
Less Changeable		

Objectives relating to behavior changes that are more changeable and more important need to be your *first* priorities. Objectives that are more important and less changeable constitute your *second* priority. The *third* priority is objectives that are less important but more changeable. Less changeable and less important objectives need to be *ignored*.

Deciding Targets

Having prioritized your objectives, make a daily list of targets that will help you accomplish the objectives selected. Since this is a daily activity, you can practice on a blank sheet of paper or make photocopies of this worksheet for repeated use.

DAY AND DATE: _____

Time	Targets

WORKSHEET 10.4

This worksheet is available online at www.pearsonhighered.com/romas.

Identifying Social Support

In each category write out the names (or initials, if you want to maintain confidentiality) of people who have helped you in the past during moments of crises.

A. Emotional Support: People Who Have Provided Love, Trust, Caring, or Empathy

Person	Support

B. Instrumental Support: People Who Have Provided Some Tangible Aid or Service

Person	Support

(continued)

Identifying Social Support (cont'd)

C. Informational Support: People Who Have Given Valuable Advice, Suggestions, and Information

Person	Support

D. Appraisal Support: People Who Have Given Useful Feedback for Self-Evaluation or Self-Reflection

Person	Support

Enhancing Effectiveness of Social Support

Reflect on the present sources of social support in your life based on Worksheet 10.4 (page 225). In the space below, complete this reflection and make a plan on enhancing the effectiveness of each level of social support.

A. Emotional Support

Quantity: _____ Adequate   _____ Inadequate

Quality: _____ Satisfactory   _____ Not Satisfactory

How will you increase and enrich emotional support?

_____

_____

B. Instrumental Support

Quantity: _____ Adequate   _____ Inadequate

Quality: _____ Satisfactory   _____ Not Satisfactory

How will you increase and enrich instrumental support?

_____

_____

C. Informational Support

Quantity: _____ Adequate   _____ Inadequate

Quality: _____ Satisfactory   _____ Not Satisfactory

How will you increase and enrich informational support?

_____

_____

D. Appraisal Support

Quantity: _____ Adequate   _____ Inadequate

Quality: _____ Satisfactory   _____ Not Satisfactory

How will you increase and enrich appraisal support?

_____

_____

Stress Management and Reduction Techniques (SMART) Practice Log

The SMART Practice Log is designed to help you experience and practice selected techniques. Record information in the SMART Practice Log for at least one week or until you have gained sufficient practice with the desired techniques. The SMART Practice Log is an application tool.

You need to self-rate the techniques that you practice in terms of their *effectiveness*, *ease of application*, and *practical utility*. Rate these criteria on a scale of 1 to 5—that is, 1 is very low; 2 is low; 3 is satisfactory; 4 is high; and 5 is very high. You may want to use the abbreviation for not applicable (NA) if you have not had enough opportunity to try the technique. Each technique has been provided with its respective worksheet number, for ready reference.

Techniques	Worksheet No.	Effectiveness	Ease of Application	Practical Utility	Reasons
A. Relaxation Techniques					
Yogic breathing, or *pranayama*	3.1	_____	_____	_____	_____
Progressive muscle relaxation	3.2	_____	_____	_____	_____
Autogenic training	3.3	_____	_____	_____	_____
Visual imagery	3.4	_____	_____	_____	_____
B. Effective Communication					
Communication assessment	4.1	_____	_____	_____	_____
Situational communication	4.2	_____	_____	_____	_____
Assessing assertive behavior	4.3	_____	_____	_____	_____
Becoming assertive	4.4	_____	_____	_____	_____

Stress Management and Reduction Techniques (SMART) Practice Log (cont'd)

Techniques	Worksheet No.	Effectiveness	Ease of Application	Practical Utility	Reasons
C. Anger Management					
Self-assessment	5.1	_____	_____	_____	_____
Managing anger	5.2	_____	_____	_____	_____
Learning active listening	5.3	_____	_____	_____	_____
D. Coping with Anxiety					
Taylor manifest anxiety scale	6.1	_____	_____	_____	_____
RET	6.2	_____	_____	_____	_____
SKY	6.3	_____	_____	_____	_____
Gestalt therapy	6.4	_____	_____	_____	_____
Systematic desensitization	6.5	_____	_____	_____	_____
E. Eating Behavior for Healthy Lifestyles					
Enhancing awareness	7.1	_____	_____	_____	_____
Balanced diet plan	7.2	_____	_____	_____	_____

(continued)

Stress Management and Reduction Techniques (SMART)
Practice Log *(cont'd)*

Techniques	Worksheet No.	Effectiveness	Ease of Application	Practical Utility	Reasons
F. Regular Physical Activity and Exercise					
Self-awareness	8.1	_____	_____	_____	_____
Target heart-raterange	8.2	_____	_____	_____	_____
Physical activity or exercise program	8.3	_____	_____	_____	_____
G. Time Management/ Financial Management					
Enhancing awareness of time	9.1	_____	_____	_____	_____
Practical steps	9.2	_____	_____	_____	_____
Financial status	9.3	_____	_____	_____	_____
H. Goals and Objectives					
Determining goals	10.1	_____	_____	_____	_____
Prioritizing objectives	10.2	_____	_____	_____	_____
Deciding targets	10.3	_____	_____	_____	_____
Identifying social support	10.4	_____	_____	_____	_____
Enhancing social support	10.5	_____	_____	_____	_____

FEEDBACK ON WORKSHEET 10.6

This worksheet has provided you with insight to determine techniques that best suit your individuality in terms of *effectiveness*, *ease of applicability*, and *practical utility*. You should also have discovered why some of the techniques are not successful for you. If these reasons are under your control, you can try to modify them. However, if these reasons are not under your control, you need to discover and practice other techniques that work. The key for success lies in consistency and determination in practicing these techniques. These techniques are more helpful in preventing and reducing stress than in managing stress. Therefore, the younger you start and incorporate these techniques, the greater the benefit will be.

Self-Agreement

I, _____ , hereby agree to practice selected techniques for stress management identified as beneficial and practical for me from the SMART Practice Log. I will not procrastinate the implementation of these techniques in my life. I will exercise regularity and self-discipline in implementing these techniques. I will periodically reward myself for this accomplishment. After attaining regularity for …

1 month, I will _____

_____ (reward)

_____

3 months, I will _____

_____ (reward)

_____

6 months, I will _____

_____ (reward)

_____

1 year, I will _____

_____ (reward)

_____

references and further readings

Addington, J. E. (1977). *All about goals and how to achieve them.* Marina del Rey, CA: DeVorss.

Alderfer, C. (1969, May). An empirical test of a new theory of human needs. *Organizational Behavioral and Human Performance,* 142–175.

Cassel, J. (1976). The contribution of the social environment to host resistance. *American Journal of Epidemiology, 104,* 107–123.

Liebler, J. G.., & McConnell, C. R. (2012. *Management principles for health professionals* (6th ed.). Sudbury, MA: Jones & Bartlett.

Green, L. G., & Kreuter, M. W. (2005). *Health promotion planning: An educational and environmental approach* (4th ed.). Boston: McGraw-Hill.

Heaney, C. A., & Israel, B. A. (2008). Social networks and social support. In K. Glanz, B. K. Rimer, & K. Viswanath (Eds.), *Health behavior and health education: Theory, research, and practice* (4th ed., pp. 189–210). San Francisco: Jossey-Bass.

House, J. S. (1981). *Work, stress, and social support.* Reading, MA: Addison-Wesley.

Kalpidou, M., Costin, D., & Morris, J. (2011). The relationship between Facebook and the well being of undergraduate college students. *Cyberpsychology, Behavior and Social Networking, 14*(4), 183–189.

Kleinke, C. L. (2002). *Coping with life challenges* (2nd ed.). Prospect Heights, IL: Waveland Press.

Mager, R. F. (1972). *Goal analysis.* Belmont, CA: Fearon Publishers/Lear Siegler.

Maslow, A. (1954). *Motivation and personality.* New York: Harper & Row.

Maslow, A. (1962). *Toward a psychology of being.* Monterey, CA: Brooks/Cole.

Prochaska, J. O., Redding, C. A., & Evers, K. E. (2008). *The transtheoretical model and stages of change.* In K. Glanz, B. K. Rimer, & K. Viswanath (Eds). *Health behavior and health education: Theory, research, and practice* (4th ed., pp. 97–122). San Francisco: Jossey-Bass.

Robbins, S. P. & Judge, T. A. (2008). *Organizational behavior* (13th ed.). Paramus, NJ: Prentice Hall.

Romas, J. A. & Zenga, D. W. (2001). *It's about change ... it's about you!* Dubuque, IA: Kendall Hunt.

Sharma, M. & Romas, J.A. (2012). *Theoretical foundations of health education and health promotion.* (2nd ed.). Sudbury, MA: Jones and Bartlett.

Guide to Pronunciation of Foreign Language Words

Abhnivesha, 6 　əbh-nē'-vāsh
Adhi, 13 　ä'-de
Adhibhotik, 6 　ädhi-bhô-tik
Adhidevik, 6 　ädhi-de-vik
Adhyatmik, 6 　ädhyät'-mik
Agna Chakra, 60 　ägna chäk'-rä
Ahankara, 6 　əhn'-kärə
Ananda, 32 　ä-nända
Asaana, 59 　äsana
Asmita, 6 　əs-mitä'
Ashtanga Yoga, 59 　ästhan yō-gə
Atharva, 6 　əth'-ərv
Atman, 6 　ätmə
Avidya, 6 　ä-vid'-yä
Ayurvedic, 6 　ä-yoor-vā'-dəc
Bhagvad Gita, 6, 127 　bhəg-vəth' gētä
Bhakti Yoga, 59 　bhäkteēyō-gə
Brahma Sutras, 6 　brəhm soō '-tra
Chakra Yoga, 59 　chäk'-rä yō-gə
Chakras, 59 　chäk'-räs
Charaka Samhita, 6 　chə-rəkə sə-nhitä'
Dharana, 59 　dhər-ənə
Dhyana, 59 　dhy-ənə
Dukha, 6 　doo-khə'
Dvesha, 6 　dväsh
Estresse, 2 　es-tress-ē
Gyana, 7 　gyä-nə
　Yoga, 59 　yō;-gə
Hatha Yoga, 59 　hath-ä yō-gə
Kama, 6 　käm
Karma Yoga, 59 　kər'-mə yō-gə
Kaya Kalpa, 60 　kə-yä kal-pa
Klesa, 6 　klā -shə
Kriya Yoga, 59–60 　krī-yä yō-gə
Kumbhaka, 58 　kumb-haka
Kundalini Shakti, 59, 60
　kun-da-lēnē shə-ktē'
Manusmriti, 6 　mà n-oō-is-mrā-*thi*
Mooladhara, 60 　mool-əd-hərə
Mudra Yoga, 59 　moō-drə yō-gə
Niyama, 59 　nī-yäm
Prajanparadha, 6 　prə-jən-pərədə'
Pranayama, 58, 59, 67, 68, 70, 228
　pränä-yâm
Pratihara, 59 　prät-i-hərə
Prosupta, 6 　prō-soō ptə
Puraka, 58 　pur-əkə'
Puranas, 6 　poo-rän
Raga, 6 　räg
Raja Yoga, 59 　rəjə yō-gə

Rechaka, 58 　rec-həkə
Relaxare, 55 　re-lax-aā e
Rig, 6 　rigg
Rinzai Zen, 60 　rin-zhäi' zhən
Sadhana, 7 　sä'-*thnä*
Sahasrara, 59, 60 　səh-əs-rar
Sama, 6 　säm
Samadhi, 7, 59 　sä-mädhi
　Bhavana, 7 　bhəv-nə
Samkhya Yoga, 6 　sän-khy yō;-gə
Shanti Yoga, 60 　shən-ti yō;-gə
Soto Zen, 60 　sō; -tō; ' zhən
Srimad Bhagvatam, 6 　shreē'-məd
　bhä-vətəm'
Stresse, 2 　stress-ē
Strictus, 2 　stric-tus
Susruta Samhita, 6
　soōsh-roō thä sə-nhitä'
Tantras, 6 　tənt'-ra
Tonu, 6 　tô-noō
Trisna, 6, 13 　trē-shnä'
Udara, 6 　oō-dər
Upanishads, 6 　upä-ni-shads
Veda(s), 6, 59 　vā'-das
　Atharva, 6 　əth'-ərv
　Rig, 6 　rigg
　Sama, 6 　säm
　Yajur, 6 　yə'-joōr
Vichchinna, 6 　vi-chinə
Vidya, 7 　vid'-yä
Yajur, 6 　yə'-joōr
Yama, 59 　yäm
Yoga, 59–60, 68 　yō;-gə
　Ashtanga, 59 　ästhan
　Bhakti, 59 　bhäktē
　Chakra, 59 　chäk'-rä
　Gyana, 59 　gyä-nə
　Hatha, 59 　hath-ä
　Karma, 59 　kər'-mə
　Kriya, 59, 60 　krī yä
　Mudra, 59 　moō-drə
　Raja, 59 　rəjə
　Shanti, 60 　shən-ti
Yogasutras, 6, 59 　yō;-gə-soō-trä
Zazen, 60 　zä-zhən
Zen, 60 　zhən
　Rinzai, 60 　rin-zhäi'
　Soto, 60 　sō-tō'
　ZA, 60 　Zä

Symbol	Key Words	Symbol	Key Words
a	asp, fat, parrot	b	bed, fable, dub, ebb
ā	ape, date, play, break, fail	d	dip, beadle, had, dodder
ä	ah, car, father, cot	f	fall, after, off, phone
		g	get, haggle, dog
e	elf, ten, berry	h	he, ahead, hotel
ē	even, meet, money, flea, grief	j	joy, agile, badge
		k	kill, tackle, bake, coat, quick
i	is, hit, mirror	l	let, yellow, ball
ī	ice, bite, high, sky	m	met, camel, trim, summer
		n	not, flannel, ton
ō	open, tone, go, boat	p	put, apple, tap
ô	all, horn, law, oar	r	red, port, dear, purr
oo	look, pull, moor, wolf	s	sell, castle, pass, nice
oo	ooze, tool, crew, rule	t	top, cattle, hat
yoo	use, cute, few	v	vat, hovel, have
yoo	cure, globule	w	will, always, sweat, quick
oi	oil, point, toy	y	yet, onion, yard
ou	out, crowd, plow	z	zebra, dazzle, haze, rise
u	up, cut, color, flood	ch	chin, catcher, arch, nature
ur	urn, fur, deter, irk	sh	she, cushion, dash, machine
		th	thin, nothing, truth
ə	a in ago	*th*	then, father, lathe
	e in agent	zh	azure, leisure, beige
	i in sanity	ŋ	ring, anger, drink
	o in comply	'	[indicates that a following]
	u in focus		or n is a syllabic consonant,
ər	perhaps, murder		as in *cattle* (kat''l), *Latin* (lat''n)

ȧ This symbol, representing the *a* in French *salle,* can best be described as intermediate between (a) and (ä).

ë This symbol represents the sound of the vowel cluster in French *coeur* and can be approximated by rounding the lips as for (ō) and pronouncing (e).

ö This symbol variously represents the sound of *eu* in French *feu* or of *ö* or *oe* in German *blöd* or *Goethe* and can be approximated by rounding the lips as for (ō) and pronouncing (ā).

ô̂ This symbol represents a range of sounds between (ô) and (u); it occurs typically in the sound of the *o* in French *tonne* or German *korrekt;* in Italian *poco* and Spanish *torero,* it is almost like English (ô), as in *horn.*

ü This symbol variously represents the sound of *u* in French *duc* and in German *grün* and can be approximated by rounding the lips as for (ō) and pronouncing (ē).

kh This symbol represents the voiceless velar or uvular fricative as in the *ch* of German *doch* or Scots English *loch.* It can be approximated by placing the tongue as for (k) but allowing the breath to escape in a stream, as in pronouncing (h).

H This symbol represents a sound similar to the preceding but formed by friction against the forward part of the palate, as in German *ich.* It can be made by placing the tongue as for English (sh) but with the tip pointing downward.

n This symbol indicates that the vowel sound immediately preceding it is nasalized; that is, the nasal passage is left open so that the breath passes through both the mouth and the nose in voicing the vowel, as in French *mon* (môn). The letter *n* itself is not pronounced unless followed by a vowel.

r This symbol represents any of various sounds used in languages other than English for the consonant *r.* It may represent the tongue-point trill or uvular trill of the *r* in French *reste* or *sur,* German *Reuter,* Italian *ricotta,* Russian *gorod,* etc.

' The apostrophe is used after final *l* and *r,* in certain French pronunciations, to indicate that they are voiceless after an unvoiced consonant, as in *lettre* (let'r'). In Russian words the "soft sign" in the Cyrillic spelling is indicated by (y'). The sound can be approximated by pronouncing an unvoiced (y) directly after the consonant involved, as in *Sevastopol* (se' väs tô̂ pəl y').

Index

List of Reviewers

We would like to thank all our reviewers, past and present, for their valuable input and contributions to this text.

GwenEllyn Anderson, *Chemeketa Community College*

Rhiannon Avery, *Boise State University*

Barbara A. Brehm Curtis, *Smith College*

Julia Carroll, *University of Houston, Clear Lake*

Richard Cavasina, *California University of Pennsylvania*

Stephen Coates-White, *South Seattle Community College*

W. Michael Felts, *East Carolina University*

Sue Fenton, *Community College of Baltimore County*

Jolynn Gardner, *University of St. Thomas*

Jim Grizzell, *California State Polytechnic University, Pomona*

Jeffrey Harris, *West Chester University*

Karen M. Hunter, *Eastern Kentucky University*

Barbara Kearney, *Murray State University*

Allen Pat Kelly, *Essex Community College*

Cathy Kennedy, *Colorado State University*

Adam Knowlden, *University of Cincinnati*

Maren Larson, *Southwest Minnesota State University*

Harlan Lee, *Bellevue Community College*

Suzanne McGowan, *Greenfield Community College*

Frances McGrath-Kovarik, *San Jose State University*

James F. McKenzie, *Ball State University*

Karen Moses, *Arizona State University*

Kristin Nesvacil, *Illinois State University*

Nancy Nygaard, *Murray State University*

Michael Olpin, *Weber State University*

William Papin, *Western Carolina University*

Glen J. Peterson, *Lakewood Community College*

Patricia Richards, *University of Idaho*

Ellen K. Rudolph, *Thomas Nelson Community College*

Glenn Schiraldi, *University of Maryland*

Kathleen Srour, *Saint Francis College*

Karen Sullivan, *Marymount University*

B.J. Wells, *Wichita State University*

Deborah A. Wuest, *Ithaca College*

Kathleen J. Zavela, *University of Northern Colorado*

Candice Zientek, *Shippensburg University*